35776003066242
615.7827 G885m 1997
Grinspoon, Lester,
Marihuana, the forbidden medicine

D0188678

Marihuana, the Forbidden Medicine

REVISED AND EXPANDED EDITION

Marihuana, the Forbidden Medicine

LESTER GRINSPOON, M.D.
AND JAMES B. BAKALAR

Yale
University
Press
New Haven
and
London

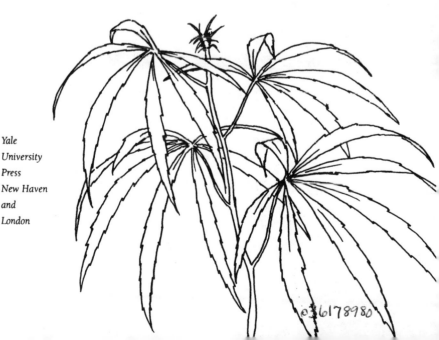

Copyright © 1997 by Yale University. All rights reserved. This book may not be reproduced, in whole or in part, including illustrations, in any form (beyond that copying permitted by Sections 107 and 108 of the U.S. Copyright Law and except by reviewers for the public press), without written permission from the publishers.

Printed in the United States of America.

Library of Congress Cataloging-in-Publication Data
Grinspoon, Lester, 1928–
Marihuana, the forbidden medicine / Lester Grinspoon and James B. Bakalar. — Rev. and exp. ed.
p.   cm.
Includes bibliographical references and index.
ISBN 978-0-300-07086-6 (pbk. : alk. paper)
1. Marijuana—Therapeutic use.   2. Marijuana—Therapeutic use—Social aspects.   3. Marijuana—Therapeutic use—Law and legislation—United States.
I. Bakalar, James B., 1943–
II. Title.
RM666.c266G75   1997
615'.7827—dc21   97-981

A catalogue record for this book is available from the British Library.

The paper in this book meets the guidelines for permanence and durability of the Committee on Production Guidelines for Book Longevity of the Council on Library Resources.

10   9

To the courageous contributors
who share their stories in this book

If there are any persons who contest a
received opinion, or who will do so if law
or opinion will let them, let us thank
them for it, open our minds to listen to
them, and rejoice that there is someone
to do for us what we otherwise ought, if
we have any regard for either the
certainty or the vitality of our
convictions, to do with much greater
labor for ourselves.
John Stuart Mill

The rejection of any source of evidence
is always treason to that ultimate rationalism
which urges forward science and philosophy alike.
Alfred North Whitehead

Contents

Preface to the Revised and
Expanded Edition   ix

Preface to the First Edition   xi

1 The History of Cannabis   1

2 Common Medical Uses   23
Cancer Chemotherapy   23
Glaucoma   45
Epilepsy   66
Multiple Sclerosis   80
Paraplegia and Quadriplegia   94
AIDS   100
Chronic Pain   109
Migraine   123
Rheumatic Diseases (Osteoarthritis and
    Ankylosing Spondylitis)   126
Pruritus   131
Premenstrual Syndrome, Menstrual Cramps,
    and Labor Pains   135
Depression and Other Mood Disorders   138

3 Less Common Medical Uses   163

Asthma   164

Insomnia   167

Other Causes of Severe Nausea   168

Antimicrobial Effects   172

Topical Anesthetic Effects   173

Antitumoral Effects   173

Dystonias   174

Adult Attention Deficit Disorder   176

Schizophrenia   178

Systemic Sclerosis (Scleroderma)   181

Crohn's Disease   186

Diabetic Gastroparesis   189

Pseudotumor Cerebri   191

Tinnitus   193

Violence   195

Post-Traumatic Stress Disorder   198

Phantom Limb Pain   200

Alcoholism and Other Addictions   202

Marihuana and Aging   214

Terminal Illness   222

4 In Defense of Anecdotal Evidence   226

5 Weighing the Risks   234

6 The Once and Future Medicine   253

Index   285

Preface to the Revised and Expanded Edition

In the years since this book was first published, it has become clear that cannabis is a remarkably versatile as well as a safe medicine. In this revised and expanded edition we have further developed the scientific and sociopolitical analysis of the prospects for acceptance of medical marihuana. We have also strengthened the case for the more common medical uses while expanding our discussion of less common uses. These assignments to more and less common categories are provisional; additional experience will provide a sounder basis for judging which medical uses are most important.

We have updated case histories where possible. Furthermore, many medical cannabis users have sought us out during the past four years to thank us and share their experiences, and some of their stories are also included in this edition. Several people have told us that the book changed their lives. One woman with multiple sclerosis, for example, said that marihuana not only relieved her muscle spasms but gave her a degree of bladder control that allowed her a new social freedom.

We are again indebted to a number of people. First we want to express our appreciation and admiration for the medical marihuana users who have shared their personal stories, whether anonymously or under their own names. Others who deserve thanks for their valuable contributions are: Ferris Boulous, Timothy Bouquet, Barry Campbell, Elizabeth Case, Dale Gieringer, Ph.D., Rick Doblin, Etienne Fontan, Betsy Grinspoon, Dave Hieshetter, Peter Barton Hutt, Tamara Jessiman, Linda LeCraw, Harry G. Levine, Timothy McGlothlin, Stich Miller, Marjorie Niland, Rosemarie O'Brien, Noreen O'Connor, Jeanne Parent, O. D. Rouse, Ed Spatz, M.D., Allen St. Pierre, Linda Payne, Steve Payne, R. Keith Stroup, Lennice Werth, and Lynn Zimmer.

Finally, we are most indebted to our assistant, Patricia Ambrose, whose good humor, limitless patience, and exceptional competence greatly enhanced our pleasure in working on this project.

Lester Grinspoon, M.D.

Preface to the First Edition

When I began to study marihuana in 1967, I had no doubt that it was a very harmful drug that was unfortunately being used by more and more foolish young people who would not listen to or could not understand the warnings about its dangers. My purpose was to define scientifically the nature and degree of those dangers. In the next three years, as I reviewed the scientific, medical, and lay literature, my views began to change. I came to understand that I, like so many other people in this country, had been brainwashed. My beliefs about the dangers of marihuana had very little empirical foundation. By the time I completed the research that formed the basis for a book, I had become convinced that cannabis was considerably less harmful than tobacco and alcohol, the most commonly used legal drugs. The book was published in 1971; its title, *Marihuana Reconsidered*, reflected my change in view.

At that time I naively believed that once people understood that marihuana was much less harmful than drugs that were already legal, they would come to favor legalization. In 1971 I confidently predicted that cannabis would be legalized for adults within the decade. I had not yet learned that there is something very special about illicit drugs. If they don't always make the drug user behave irrationally, they certainly cause many non-users to behave that way. Instead of making marihuana legally available to adults, we have continued to criminalize many millions of Americans. About 300,000 mostly young people are arrested on marihuana charges each year, and the political climate has now deteriorated to the point where it has become difficult to discuss marihuana openly and freely. It could almost be said that there is a climate of psychopharmacological McCarthyism.

One indication of this climate is the rise in mandatory drug testing, which is analogous to the loyalty oaths of the McCarthy era. Hardly anyone believed that forced loyalty oaths would enhance national security, but people who refused to take such oaths risked loss of their jobs and reputations. Today we are witnessing the imposition of a chemical loyalty oath. Mandatory, often random testing of urine samples for the presence of illicit drugs is increasingly demanded as a condition of employment. People who test positive may be fired or, if they wish to keep their jobs, may be involuntarily assigned to drug counseling or "employee assistance" programs.

All this is of little use in preventing or treating drug abuse. In the case of cannabis, urine testing can easily be defeated by chemical alteration of the urine or substitution of someone else's urine. Even if the urine sample has not been altered, the available tests are far from perfect. The cheaper ones are seriously inaccurate, and even the more expensive and accurate ones are fallible because of laboratory error and passive exposure to marihuana smoke. But even an infallible test would be of little use in preventing or treating drug abuse. Marihuana metabolites (breakdown products) remain in the urine for days after a single exposure and for weeks after a long-term user stops. Their presence bears no established relationship to drug effects on the brain. It tells little about when the drug was used, how much was used, or what effects it had or has. Like loyalty oaths imposed on government employees, urine testing for marihuana is useless for its ostensible purpose. It is little more than shotgun harassment designed to impose outward conformity.

Another aspect of psychopharmacological McCarthyism is suggested by the response to a publication in the May 1990 issue of *American Psychologist*. Two psychologists at the University of California, Berkeley, reported the results of a rigorous longitudinal study of 101 eighteen-year-olds whom they had been following since the age of five to examine the relation between psychological characteristics and drug use. The results showed that adolescents who had engaged in some drug experimentation (mainly with marihuana) were the best adjusted. The authors comment:

> Adolescents who used drugs frequently were maladjusted, show- ing a distinct personality syndrome marked by interpersonal alienation, poor impulse control, and manifest emotional dis- tress. Adolescents who had never experimented with any drug were relatively anxious, emotionally constricted, and lacking in social skills. Psychological differences between frequent drug users, experimenters, and abstainers could be traced to the earli- est years of childhood and related to the quality of their parent- ing. The findings indicate that (a) problem drug use is a symp- tom, not a cause, of personal and social maladjustment, and (b) the meaning of drug use can be understood only in the context of an individual's personality structure and developmental history.[1]

This study suggests that the current anti-drug campaign ("Just Say No") is misguided because it concentrates on symptoms rather than underlying problems.

A hue and cry began immediately. The director of a San Francisco drug prevention program said that it was irresponsible for researchers to report that "dabbling with drugs was 'not necessarily catastrophic' for some youths and may simply be a part of normal adolescent ex- perimentation." A physician who directs the adolescent recovery cen- ter of a metropolitan hospital asked, "What does this do to the kids who made a commitment to be abstinent? Now they're being told they're a bunch of dorks and geeks. You can imagine how much more peer pressure is going to be put on them." An author writing in *Pride Quarterly* (Summer 1990) stated: "Based on the experiences of only

---

1. J. Shedler and J. Block, "Adolescent Drug Use and Psychological Health: A Longi- tudinal Inquiry," *American Psychologist* 45 (May 1990): 612–630.

101 subjects, all living in San Francisco, the study drew national attention due to its outrageous conclusion." "Unfortunately," continued the writer, "the permissive thinking which surfaced in the California study will continue to exist in the United States until truly effective drug education reaches beyond the elementary classroom. However, too few educators themselves have seen the latest discoveries about the health consequences of drug use."[2] It was all reminiscent of Stalinist party-line criticism of science.

In spite of the illegality of marihuana and the prejudices against it, large numbers of Americans continue to use cannabis regularly. Once considered a youthful indulgence or expression of youthful rebellion, marihuana smoking is now a common adult practice. Millions have smoked marihuana for years, and many of them will continue to smoke it for the rest of their lives. They are convinced that they are harming no one else and not harming themselves, if at all, as much as cigarette smokers or alcohol drinkers are.

Most users, in fact, believe that marihuana enhances their lives—a subject rarely discussed in print. In more than two decades of research, I have read a great deal about the potential harmfulness of cannabis (much of it nonsense) and very little about its value. Although this value has several aspects, medical use is one of the most important and one that has been seriously neglected. I have come to conclude that if any other drug had revealed similar therapeutic promise combined with a similar record of safety, professionals and the public would have shown far more interest in it. The largely undeserved reputation of cannabis as a harmful recreational drug and the resulting legal restrictions have made medical use and research difficult. As a result, the medical community has become ignorant about cannabis and has been both a victim and an agent in the spread of misinformation and frightening myths.

What follows is largely a book of stories, because most of the evidence on marihuana's medical properties is anecdotal. Some day the

2. J. Diaz, "Furor over Report of Teenage Drug Use," *San Francisco Chronicle*, May 15, 1990; *Pride Quarterly* (Atlanta), Summer 1990, pp. 1, 8.

systematic neglect of the research community will be remedied and the authors of a book on the medical uses of marihuana will be able to review a large clinical literature. James Bakalar and I hope to reverse prejudices, relieve ignorance, and help prepare the way for that research by exploring the known and potential therapeutic uses of this remarkable substance.

This is a book by two authors and many contributors. Most of the contributors were recruited by word of mouth or by referral, but some came to our attention through testimony they gave before Drug Enforcement Agency Administrative Law Judge Francis Young during the 1986 hearings on the rescheduling of marihuana. Robert Randall and Alice O'Leary of the Alliance for Cannabis Therapeutics helped us locate some of these patients. We are indebted to Kevin Zeese of the Drug Policy Foundation for, among other things, providing us with a transcript of the hearings. Our manuscript benefited immensely from critical readings by Kenneth Arndt, M.D., Ann Druyan, John Gehring, M.D., David and Betsy Grinspoon, Norman Jaffe, M.D., Simeon Locke, M.D., Susan F. Milmoe, Carl Sagan, Richard Schultes, and Arnold S. Trebach. Our project was also aided in diverse ways by Peggy S. Alcorn, Beth Banov, Del Cogswell Brebner, Elizabeth Case, Leslie Druyan, Paul Geissler, James Johnson, Jeff Moore, June Riedlinger, Alexander Shulgin, Lewis L. Van Hoosear, M.D., and Lennice Werth.

Lester Grinspoon, M.D.

Marihuana,
the Forbidden
Medicine

1 The History of Cannabis

The marihuana, cannabis, or hemp plant is one of the oldest psychoactive plants known to humanity. Botanically it is classified as belonging to the family Cannabaceae and the genus *Cannabis*. Most botanists agree that there are three species: *Cannabis sativa*, the most widespread of the three, is tall, gangly, and loosely branched, growing as high as twenty feet; *Cannabis indica* is shorter, about three or four feet high, pyramidal in shape, and densely branched; *Cannabis ruderalis* is about two feet high with few or no branches. There are also differences among these species in the leaves, stems, and resin. According to an alternative classification, the genus has only one highly variable species, *Cannabis sativa*, with two subspecies, *sativa* and *indica*. The first is more northerly and produces more fiber and oil; the second is more southerly and produces more of the intoxicating resin.

Cannabis has become one of the most widespread and diversified of plants. It grows as a weed and cultivated plant all over the world in a variety of climates and soils. The fiber has been used for cloth and paper and was the most important source of rope until the development of synthetic fibers. The seeds (or, strictly speaking, akenes—small hard fruits) have been used as bird feed and sometimes as human food. The oil contained in the seeds was once used for lighting and soap and is now sometimes employed in the manufacture of varnish, linoleum, and artists' paints.

The chemical compounds responsible for the intoxicating and medicinal effects are found mainly in a sticky golden resin exuded from the flowers on the female plants. The function of the resin is thought to be protection from heat and preservation of moisture during reproduction. The plants highest in resin therefore grow in hot regions like Mexico, the Middle East, and India. When the reproductive process is over and the fruits are fully ripe, no more resin is secreted.

The cannabis preparations used in India often serve as a folk standard of potency. The three varieties are known as *bhang, ganja,* and *charas.* The least potent and cheapest preparation, bhang, is produced from the dried and crushed leaves, seeds, and stems. Ganja, prepared from the flowering tops of cultivated female plants, is two or three times as strong as bhang; the difference is somewhat akin to the difference between beer and fine Scotch. Charas is the pure resin, also known as hashish in the Middle East. Any of these preparations can be smoked, eaten, or mixed in drinks. The marihuana used in the United States is equivalent to bhang or, increasingly in the past two decades, to ganja.

The marihuana plant contains more than 460 known compounds, of which more than 60 have the 21-carbon structure typical of cannabinoids. The only cannabinoid that is both highly psychoactive and present in large amounts, usually 1–5 percent by weight, is (-)3,4-trans-delta-1-tetrahydrocannabinol, also known as delta-1-THC, delta-9-THC, or simply THC. A few other tetrahydrocannabinols are about as potent as delta-9-THC but are present in only a few varieties of cannabis and in much smaller quantities. A number of synthetic congeners (chemical relatives) of THC have been developed under such names as synhexyl, nabilone, and levonatradol. The other two major types of cannabinoid are the cannabidiols and the cannabinols. It appears that the plant first produces the mildly active cannabidiols, which are converted to tetrahydrocannabinols and then broken down to relatively inactive cannabinols as the plant matures.

In 1990 researchers identified nerve receptors in the brain that are stimulated by THC and cloned the gene that gives rise to those receptors. In 1992 the natural body chemical that binds to those receptors was identified. It has been named anandamide, after a Sanskrit word meaning "bliss."[1] Receptors for anandamide (and THC) are located mainly in the cerebral cortex and in the basal ganglia and cerebellum, parts of the brain associated with body movements. The receptors in the cortex may explain the cognitive effects of cannabis, and those found in the basal ganglia and cerebellum may account for its effects on muscle spasms and other body movement disorders.

A native of central Asia, cannabis may have been cultivated as much as ten thousand years ago. It was certainly cultivated in China by 4000 B.C. and in Turkestan by 3000 B.C. It has long been used as a medicine in India, China, the Middle East, Southeast Asia, South Africa, and South America. The first evidence of the medicinal use of cannabis is an herbal published during the reign of the Chinese Emperor Chen Nung five thousand years ago. It was recommended for malaria, constipation, rheumatic pains, "absentmindedness," and "female disorders." Another Chinese herbalist recommended a mixture of hemp, resin, and wine as an analgesic during surgery. In India cannabis has been recommended to quicken the mind, lower fevers, induce sleep, cure dysentery, stimulate appetite, improve digestion, relieve headaches, and cure venereal disease. In Africa it was used for dysentery, malaria, and other fevers. Today certain tribes treat snakebite with hemp or smoke it before childbirth. Hemp was also noted as a remedy by Galen and other physicians of the classical and Hellenistic eras, and it was highly valued in medieval Europe. The English clergyman Robert Burton, in his famous work *The Anatomy of Melancholy*, published in 1621, suggested the use of cannabis in the treatment of depression. The *New English Dispensatory* of 1764 recommended applying hemp roots to the skin for inflammation, a remedy that was already popular in eastern Europe. The *Edinburgh New Dispensary* of 1794 included a long description of the effects of hemp

1. L. A. Matsuda, S. J. Lolait, M. J. Brownstein, A. C. Young, and T. I. Bonner, "Structure of a Cannabinoid Receptor and Functional Expression of the Cloned cDNA," *Nature* 346 (Aug. 9, 1990): 561–564. W. Devane, L. Hanus, A. Breuer, et al., "Isolation and Structure of a Brain Constituent that Binds to the Cannabinoid Receptor," *Science* 258 (Dec. 18, 1992): 1946–1948.

and stated that the oil was useful in the treatment of coughs, vene-real disease, and urinary incontinence. A few years later the physician Nicholas Culpeper summarized all the conditions for which cannabis was supposed to be medically useful.

But in the West cannabis did not come into its own as a medicine until the mid-nineteenth century. During its heyday, from 1840 to 1900, more than one hundred papers were published in the Western medical literature recommending it for various illnesses and discomforts.[2] It could almost be said that physicians of a century ago knew more about cannabis than contemporary physicians do; certainly they were more interested in exploring its therapeutic potential.

The first Western physician to take an interest in cannabis as a medicine was W. B. O'Shaughnessy, a young professor at the Medical College of Calcutta, who had observed its use in India. He gave cannabis to animals, satisfied himself that it was safe, and began to use it with patients suffering from rabies, rheumatism, epilepsy, and tetanus. In a report published in 1839, he wrote that he had found tincture of hemp (a solution of cannabis in alcohol, taken orally) to be an an effective analgesic. He was also impressed with its muscle-relaxant properties and called it "an anticonvulsive remedy of the greatest value."[3]

O'Shaughnessy returned to England in 1842 and provided cannabis to pharmacists. Doctors in Europe and the United States soon began to prescribe it for a variety of physical conditions. Cannabis was even given to Queen Victoria by her court physician. It was listed in the United States Dispensatory in 1854 (with a warning that large doses were dangerous and that it was a powerful "narcotic"). Commercial cannabis preparations could be bought in drugstores. During the Centennial Exposition of 1876 in Philadelphia, some pharmacists carried ten pounds or more of hashish.[4]

2. T. H. Mikuriya, ed., *Marijuana: Medical Papers, 1839–1972* (Oakland: Medi-Comp, 1973).

3. W. B. O'Shaughnessy, "On the Preparations of the Indian Hemp, or gunjah (Cannabis indica): The Effects on the Animal System in Health, and Their Utility in the Treatment of Tetanus and Other Convulsive Diseases," *Transactions of the Medical and Physical Society of Bengal* (1838–1840): 421–461.

4. E. L. Abel, *Marihuana: The First Twelve Thousand Years* (New York: Plenum, 1980).

Meanwhile, reports on cannabis accumulated in the medical literature. In 1860 Dr. R. R. M'Meens reported the findings of the Committee on Cannabis Indica to the Ohio State Medical Society.[5] After
acknowledging a debt to O'Shaughnessy, M'Meens reviewed symptoms and conditions for which Indian hemp had been found useful,
including tetanus, neuralgia, dysmenorrhea (painful menstruation),
convulsions, the pain of rheumatism and childbirth, asthma, post-
partum psychosis, gonorrhea, and chronic bronchitis. As a hypnotic
(sleep-inducing drug) he compared it to opium: "Its effects are less
intense, and the secretions are not so much suppressed by it. Digestion is not disturbed; the appetite rather increased; . . . The whole
effect of hemp being less violent, and producing a more natural sleep,
without interfering with the actions of the internal organs, it is certainly often preferable to opium, although it is not equal to that drug
in strength and reliability." Like O'Shaughnessy, M'Meens emphasized
the remarkable capacity of cannabis to stimulate appetite.

Interest persisted into the next generation. In 1887, H. A. Hare ex-
tolled the capacity of hemp to subdue restlessness and anxiety and
distract a patient's mind in terminal illness. In these circumstances, he
wrote, "The patient, whose most painful symptom has been mental
trepidation, may become more happy or even hilarious." He believed
cannabis to be as effective a pain reliever as opium: "During the time
that this remarkable drug is relieving pain, a very curious psychical
condition sometimes manifests itself; namely, that the diminution of
the pain seems to be due to its fading away in the distance, so that
the pain becomes less and less, just as the pain in a delicate ear would
grow less and less as a beaten drum was carried farther and farther
out of the range of hearing."[6] Hare also noted that hemp is an excellent topical anesthetic, especially for the mucous membranes of the
mouth and tongue—a property well known to dentists in the nineteenth century.

In 1890, J. R. Reynolds, a British physician, summarized thirty years

5. R. R. M'Meens, "Report of the Committee on Cannabis Indica," *Transactions,* Fif-
teenth Annual Meeting of the Ohio State Medical Society, Columbus, 1860.

6. H. A. Hare, "Clinical and Physiological Notes on the Action of Cannabis indica,"
Therapeutic Gazette 11 (1887): 225–226.

of experience with Cannabis indica, recommending it for patients with "senile insomnia": "In this class of cases I have found nothing comparable in utility to a moderate dose of Indian hemp." According to Reynolds, hemp remained effective for months and even years without an increase in the dose. He also found it valuable in the treatment of various forms of neuralgia, including tic douloureux (a painful facial neurological disorder), and added that it was useful in preventing migraine attacks: "Very many victims of this malady have for years kept their suffering in abeyance by taking hemp at the moment of threatening or onset of the attack." He also found it useful for certain kinds of epilepsy, for depression, and sometimes for asthma and dysmenorrhea.[7]

Doctor J. B. Mattison, urging physicians to continue using hemp, in 1891 called it "a drug that has a special value in some morbid conditions and the intrinsic merit and safety of which entitles it to a place it once held in therapeutics." Mattison reviewed its uses as an analgesic and hypnotic, with special reference to dysmenorrhea, chronic rheumatism, asthma, gastric ulcer, and morphine addiction, but for him the most important use of cannabis was in treating "that opprobrium of the healing art—migraine." Reviewing his own and earlier physicians' experiences, he concluded that cannabis not only blocks the pain of migraine but prevents migraine attacks.[8] Years later William Osler expressed his agreement, saying that cannabis was "probably the most satisfactory remedy" for migraine.[9]

Mattison's report concluded on a wistful note:

> Dr. Suckling wrote me: "The young men rarely prescribe it." To them I specially commend it. With a wish for speedy effect, it is so easy to use that modern mischief maker, hypodermic morphia,

7. J. R. Reynolds, "Therapeutic Uses and Toxic Effects of Cannabis indica," Lancet 1 (1890): 637.

8. J. B. Mattison, "Cannabis indica as an Anodyne and Hypnotic," St. Louis Medical Surgical Journal 61 (1891): 266–267.

9. W. Osler, The Principles and Practice of Medicine, 8th ed. (New York: Appleton, 1913), 1089.

that they [young physicians] are prone to forget remote results of incautious opiate giving.

Would that the wisdom which has come to their professional fathers through, it may be, a hapless experience might serve them to steer clear of narcotic shoals on which many a patient has gone awreck.

Indian hemp is not here lauded as a specific. It will, at times, fail. So do other drugs. But the many cases in which it acts well entitle it to a large and lasting confidence.[10]

As he noted, the medical use of cannabis was already in decline by 1890. The potency of cannabis preparations was too variable, and individual responses to orally ingested cannabis seemed erratic and unpredictable. Another reason for the neglect of research on the analgesic properties of cannabis was that the greatly increased use of opiates after the invention of the hypodermic syringe in the 1850s allowed soluble drugs to be injected for fast relief of pain; hemp products are insoluble in water and so cannot easily be administered by injection. Toward the end of the nineteenth century, the development of such synthetic drugs as aspirin, chloral hydrate, and barbiturates, which are chemically more stable than *Cannabis indica* and therefore more reliable, hastened the decline of cannabis as a medicine. But the new drugs had striking disadvantages. More than a thousand people die from aspirin-induced bleeding each year in the United States, and barbiturates are, of course, far more dangerous. One might have expected physicians looking for better analgesics and hypnotics to turn to cannabinoid substances, especially after 1940, when it became possible to study congeners (chemical relatives) of THC that might have more stable and specific effects.

But the Marihuana Tax Act of 1937 undermined any such experimentation. This law was the culmination of a campaign organized by the Federal Bureau of Narcotics under Harry Anslinger in which the public was led to believe that marihuana was addictive and that its use

10. Mattison, "*Cannabis indica* as Anodyne," 271.

led to violent crimes, psychosis, and mental deterioration. The film *Reefer Madness*, made as part of Anslinger's campaign, may be a joke to the sophisticated today, but it was once regarded as a serious attempt to address a social problem, and the atmosphere and attitudes it exemplified and promoted continue to influence our culture today.

Under the Marihuana Tax Act, anyone using the hemp plant for certain defined industrial or medical purposes was required to register and pay a tax of a dollar an ounce. A person using marihuana for any other purpose had to pay a tax of $100 an ounce on unregistered transactions. Those who failed to comply were subject to large fines or prison for tax evasion. The law was not directly aimed at the medical use of marihuana—its purpose was to discourage recreational marihuana smoking. It was put in the form of a revenue measure to evade the effect of Supreme Court decisions that reserved to the states the right to regulate most commercial transactions. By forcing some marihuana transactions to be registered and others to be taxed heavily, the government could make it prohibitively expensive to obtain the drug legally for any other than medical purposes. Almost incidentally, the law made medical use of cannabis difficult because of the extensive paperwork required of doctors who wanted to use it. The Federal Bureau of Narcotics followed up with "anti-diversion" regulations that contributed to physicians' disenchantment. Cannabis was removed from the United States Pharmacopoeia and National Formulary in 1941.

A reading of the hearings in which the bill was examined by the House Ways and Means Committee before its passage shows how little data supported the judgment that marihuana was harmful and how much mass hysteria surrounded the subject. The only dissident witness was W. C. Woodward, a physician-lawyer serving as legislative counsel for the American Medical Association. He supported the aims of Congress but tried to persuade it to enact less restrictive legislation, on the ground that future investigators might discover substantial medical uses for cannabis. In reference to marihuana "addiction," Woodward commented:

The newspapers have called attention to it so prominently that there must be some grounds for their statements. It has surprised me, however, that the facts on which these statements have been based have not been brought before this committee by competent primary evidence. We are referred to newspaper publications concerning the prevalence of marihuana addiction. We are told that the use of marihuana causes crime.

But as yet no one has been produced from the Bureau of Prisons to show the number of prisoners who have been found addicted to the marihuana habit. An informal inquiry shows that the Bureau of Prisons has no evidence on that point.

You have been told that school children are great users of marihuana cigarettes. No one has been summoned from the Children's Bureau to show the nature and extent of the habit among children.

Inquiry of the Children's Bureau shows that they have had no occasion to investigate it and know nothing particularly of it.

Inquiry of the Office of Education—and they certainly should know something of the prevalence of the habit among the school children of the county, if there is a prevalence of the habit—indicates that they have had no occasion to investigate and know nothing of it.[11]

Congressmen questioned Woodward closely and critically about his educational background, his relationship to the American Medical Association, and his views on medical legislation of the previous fifteen years. His objections to the quality and sources of the evidence against cannabis did not endear him to the legislators. Representative John Dingell's questions are typical:

Mr. Dingell: We know that it is a habit that is spreading, particularly among youngsters. We learn that from the pages of the news-

11. U.S. Congress, House Ways and Means Committee, Hearings on H.R. 6385: Taxation of Marihuana, 75th Cong., 1st sess., Apr. 27, 1937, 91, 94.

papers. You say that Michigan has a law regulating it. We have a State Law, but we do not seem to be able to get anywhere with it, because, as I have said, the habit is growing. The number of victims is increasing each year.

Dr. *Woodward:* There is no evidence of that.

Mr. *Dingell:* I have not been impressed by your testimony here as reflecting the sentiment of the high-class members of the medical profession in my State. I am confident that the medical profession in the State of Michigan, and in Wayne County particularly, or in my district, will subscribe wholeheartedly to any law that will suppress this thing, despite the fact that there is a $1 tax imposed.

Dr. *Woodward:* If there was any law that would absolutely suppress the thing, perhaps that is true, but when the law simply contains provisions that impose a useless expense, and does not accomplish the result—

Mr. *Dingell* (interposing): That is simply your personal opinion. That is kindred to the opinion you entertained with reference to the Harrison Narcotics Act.

Dr. *Woodward:* If we had been asked to cooperate in drafting it—

Mr. *Dingell* (interposing): You are not cooperating in drafting this at all.

Dr. *Woodward:* As a matter of fact, it does not serve to suppress the use of opium and cocaine.

Mr. *Dingell:* The medical profession should be doing its utmost to aid in the suppression of this curse that is eating the very vitals of the Nation.

Dr. *Woodward:* They are.

Mr. *Dingell:* Are you not simply piqued because you were not consulted in the drafting of the bill? [12]

Woodward was finally cut off with the admonition: "You are not cooperative in this. If you want to advise us on legislation you ought to come here with some constructive proposals rather than criticisms, rather than trying to throw obstacles in the way of something that the

12. Ibid., 116.

Federal Government is trying to do."[13] His testimony was futile. The bill became law on October 1, 1937. Many state laws, just as punitive and hastily conceived, followed.

One of the few public officials who responded rationally to the marihuana issue in the 1930s was New York's Mayor Fiorello La-Guardia. In 1938 he appointed a committee of scientists to study the medical, sociological, and psychological aspects of marihuana use in New York City. Two internists, three psychiatrists, two pharmacologists, a public health expert, the commissioners of Correction, Health, and Hospitals, and the director of the Division of Psychiatry of the Department of Hospitals made up the committee. They began their study in 1940 and presented detailed findings in 1944 under the title "The Marihuana Problem in the City of New York." This largely disregarded study dispelled many of the myths that had spurred passage of the Tax Act. The Committee found no proof that major crime was associated with marihuana or that it caused aggressive or antisocial behavior; marihuana was not sexually overstimulating and did not change personality; there was no evidence of acquired tolerance.

In September 1942 the *American Journal of Psychiatry* published "The Psychiatric Aspects of Marihuana Intoxication," by two of the New York study's investigators, Samuel Allentuck and Karl M. Bowman. Among other things, Allentuck and Bowman wrote that habituation to cannabis is not as strong as habituation to tobacco or alcohol. Three months later, in December, an editorial in the *Journal of the American Medical Association* described Allentuck and Bowman's article as "a careful study" and mentioned potential therapeutic uses of cannabis in the treatment of depression, appetite loss, and opiate addiction.

In the next few years that journal's editors were induced to change their minds under government pressure. They received and published letters denouncing the LaGuardia report from Harry Anslinger in January 1943 and from R. J. Bouquet, an expert working for the Nar-

13. Ibid., 117.

cotics Commission of the League of Nations, in April 1944. Finally, the American Medical Association expressed its agreement with the Federal Bureau of Narcotics in an editorial in April 1945:

> For many years medical scientists have considered cannabis a dangerous drug. Nevertheless, a book called *Marihuana Problems* by the New York City Mayor's Committee on Marihuana submits an analysis by seventeen doctors of tests on 77 prisoners and, on this narrow and thoroughly unscientific foundation, draws sweeping and inadequate conclusions which minimize the harmfulness of marihuana. Already the book has done harm. . . . The book states unqualifiedly to the public that the use of this narcotic does not lead to physical, mental or moral degeneration and that permanent deleterious effects from its continued use were not observed on 77 prisoners. This statement has already done great damage to the cause of law enforcement. Public officials will do well to disregard this unscientific, uncritical study, and continue to regard marihuana as a menace wherever it is purveyed.

In the words of R. S. deRopp, the journal had "abandoned its customary restraint and voiced its editorial wrath in scolding tones. So fierce was the editorial that one might suppose that the learned members of the mayor's committee . . . had formed some unhallowed league with the 'tea-pad' proprietors [owners of places where marihuana users gathered to smoke] to undermine the city's health by deliberately misrepresenting the facts about marihuana."[14] For more than forty years after that editorial, the American Medical Association steadfastly maintained a position on marihuana closely allied to that of the Federal Bureau of Narcotics and its successor agencies. The

---

14. S. Allentuck and K. M. Bowman, "The Psychiatric Aspects of Marihuana Intoxication," *American Journal of Psychiatry* 99 (1942): 248–251; Editorial: "Recent Investigation of Marihuana," *Journal of the American Medical Association* (hereafter *JAMA*) 120 (1942): 1128–1129; Letter: Anslinger, "The Psychiatric Aspects of Marihuana Intoxication," *JAMA* 121 (1943): 212–213; Letter: Bouquet, "Marihuana Intoxication," *JAMA* 124 (1944): 1010–1011; Editorial: "Marihuana Problems," *JAMA* 127 (1945): 1129; R. S. deRopp, *Drugs and the Mind* (New York: St. Martin's, 1957), 108–109.

published statements of its Council on Mental Health have too often been contributions to the misinformation and frightening mythology that surround the marihuana issue.

Although virtually no medical investigation of cannabis was conducted for many years, the government did not entirely lose interest. Shortly after one of us (L.G.) published a book on marihuana in 1971, a chemist who had read it told us that his employer, the Arthur D. Little Company, had been given millions of dollars in government contracts to identify military uses for cannabis. He said that they had found none but had come across several important therapeutic leads. He visited us to discuss the economic feasibility of developing cannabinoid congeners commercially, but he could not give us the evidence because it was classified.

In the 1960s, as large numbers of people began to use marihuana recreationally, anecdotes about its medical utility began to appear, generally not in the medical literature but in the form of letters to popular magazines like Playboy. Meanwhile, legislative concern about recreational use increased, and in 1970 Congress passed the Comprehensive Drug Abuse Prevention and Control Act (also called the Controlled Substances Act), which assigned psychoactive drugs to five schedules and placed cannabis in Schedule I, the most restrictive. According to the legal definition, Schedule I drugs have no medical use and a high potential for abuse, and they cannot be used safely even under a doctor's supervision. By that time the renaissance of interest in cannabis as a medicine was already well under way. Two years later, in 1972, the National Organization for the Reform of Marijuana Laws (NORML) petitioned the Bureau of Narcotics and Dangerous Drugs (formerly the Federal Bureau of Narcotics) to transfer marihuana to Schedule II so that it could be legally prescribed by physicians. As the legal proceedings have continued, other parties have joined, including the Drug Policy Foundation and the Physicians' Association for AIDS Care.

The hearings before the Bureau of Narcotics and Dangerous Drugs (BNDD) were instructive. As one of us (L. G.) waited to testify on the medical uses of cannabis, he witnessed the effort to place pentazocine

(Talwin), a synthetic opioid analgesic made by Winthrop Pharmaceuticals, on the schedule of dangerous drugs. The testimony indicated several hundred cases of addiction, a number of overdose deaths, and considerable evidence of abuse. Six lawyers from the drug company, briefcases in hand, came forward to prevent the classification of pentazocine, or at least ensure that it was placed in one of the less restrictive schedules. They succeeded in part; it became a Schedule IV drug, available by prescription with minor restrictions. In the testimony on cannabis, the next drug to be considered, there was no evidence of overdose deaths or addiction—simply many witnesses, both patients and physicians, testifying to its medical utility. The government refused to transfer it to Schedule II. Might the outcome have been different if a large drug company with enormous financial resources had a commercial interest in cannabis?

In rejecting the NORML petition, the Bureau of Narcotics and Dangerous Drugs failed to call for public hearings, as required by law. The reason it gave was that reclassification would violate U.S. treaty obligations under the United Nations Single Convention on Narcotic Substances. NORML responded in January 1974 by filing a suit against the BNDD. The U.S. Second Circuit Court of Appeals reversed the bureau's dismissal of the petition, remanding the case for reconsideration and criticizing both the bureau and the Department of Justice. In September 1975, the Drug Enforcement Administration (DEA), successor to the BNDD, acknowledged that treaty obligations did not prevent the rescheduling of marihuana but continued to refuse public hearings. NORML again filed suit. In October 1980, after much further legal maneuvering, the Court of Appeals remanded the NORML petition to the DEA for reconsideration for the third time. The government reclassified synthetic delta-9-THC (dronabinol) as a Schedule II drug in 1985 but kept marihuana itself—and the THC derived from marihuana—in Schedule I. Finally, in May 1986, the DEA Administrator announced the public hearings ordered by the court seven years earlier.

Those hearings began in the summer of 1986 and lasted two years. The parties that sought rescheduling were NORML, a membership-funded educational organization, founded in 1970, which opposes all criminal prohibitions against marihuana and marihuana smoking; the Alliance for Cannabis Therapeutics, a nonprofit organization founded in 1980 to make marihuana available by prescription; the Cannabis Corporation of America, a pharmaceutical firm established with the intention of extracting natural cannabinoids for therapeutic use when cannabis is placed in Schedule II; and the Ethiopian Zion Coptic Church, which considers marihuana a sacred plant essential to its religious rituals. These groups were opposed by the DEA, the International Chiefs of Police, and the National Federation of Parents for Drug-Free Youth, another membership-funded educational organization.

The lengthy hearings involved many witnesses, including both patients and doctors, and thousands of pages of documentation. The record of these hearings constitutes the most extensive recent exploration of the evidence on cannabis as a medicine. Administrative law judge Francis L. Young reviewed the evidence and rendered his decision on September 6, 1988. Young said that approval by a "significant minority" of physicians was enough to meet the standard of "currently accepted medical use in treatment in the United States" established by the Controlled Substances Act for a Schedule II drug. He added that "marihuana, in its natural form, is one of the safest therapeutically active substances known to man. . . . One must reasonably conclude that there is accepted safety for use of marihuana under medical supervision. To conclude otherwise, on the record, would be unreasonable, arbitrary, and capricious." Young went on to recommend "that the Administrator [of the DEA] conclude that the marihuana plant considered as a whole has a currently accepted medical use in treatment in the United States, that there is no lack of accepted safety for use of it under medical supervision and that it may lawfully be transferred from Schedule I to Schedule II."[15]

In determining what "currently accepted medical use" meant for

15. Drug Enforcement Administration (hereafter DEA), In the Matter of Marijuana Rescheduling Petition, Docket 86–22, Opinion, Recommended Ruling, Findings of Fact, Conclusions of Law, and Decision of Administrative Law Judge, Sept. 6, 1988.

legal purposes, Judge Young was adopting the view of the petitioners and rejecting that of the DEA, whose criteria were the result of a previous legal challenge involving the drug 3,4-methylenedioxymethamphetamine (MDMA). In 1984 the DEA placed this previously unscheduled drug in Schedule I. The placement was challenged by a group of physicians and others who believed that MDMA had therapeutic potential. After extensive hearings, the administrative law judge rejected the DEA's position that MDMA had no accepted medical use in treatment in the United States and agreed with the challengers that it should be placed in Schedule III rather than Schedule I. The DEA administrator rejected this recommendation. The challengers appealed to the U.S. First Circuit Court of Appeals, which ruled in their favor, finding that formal approval for marketing by the Food and Drug Administration, the DEA's criterion for "accepted medical use in treatment in the United States," was unacceptable under the terms of the Controlled Substances Act.[16]

The DEA administrator responded with the following new criteria for accepted medical use of a drug: (1) scientifically determined and accepted knowledge of its chemistry; (2) scientific knowledge of its toxicology and pharmacology in animals; (3) effectiveness in human beings established through scientifically designed clinical trials; (4) general availability of the substance and information about its use; (5) recognition of its clinical use in generally accepted pharmacopoeia, medical references, journals, or textbooks; (6) specific indications for the treatment of recognized disorders; (7) recognition of its use by organizations or associations of physicians; and (8) recognition and use by a substantial segment of medical practitioners in the United States. These were the criteria rejected by Judge Young in his marihuana decision.

The DEA disregarded the opinion of its own administrative law judge and refused to reschedule marihuana. The agency's lawyer remarked, "The judge seems to hang his hat on what he calls a respectable minority of physicians. What percent are you talking about? One

16. Grinspoon v. DEA, 828 F.2d 881 (1st Cir. 1987).

half of one percent? One quarter of one percent?" DEA Administrator John Lawn went further, calling claims for the medical utility of marihuana a "dangerous and cruel hoax."[17] In March 1991 the plaintiffs appealed yet again, and in April the District of Columbia Court of Appeals unanimously ordered the DEA to reexamine its standards, suggesting that they were illogical and that marihuana could never satisfy them. An illegal drug could not be used by a substantial number of doctors or cited as a remedy in medical texts. As the court pointed out, "We are hard pressed to understand how one could show that any Schedule I drug was in general use or generally available."[18] The court returned the case to the DEA for further explanation, but it offered no direct challenge to the central dogma that marihuana lacks therapeutic value. The DEA issued a final rejection of all pleas for reclassification in March 1992.

Despite the obstructionism of the federal government, a few patients have been able to obtain marihuana legally for therapeutic purposes. State governments began to respond in a limited way to pressure from patients and physicians in the 1970s. In 1978, New Mexico enacted the first law designed to make marihuana available for medical use. Thirty-three states followed in the late 1970s and early 1980s.[19] In 1992, Massachusetts became the thirty-fourth state to enact such legislation, and in 1994 Missouri became the thirty-fifth.

But the laws proved difficult to implement. Because marihuana is not recognized as a medicine under federal law, states can dispense it only by establishing formal research programs and getting FDA approval for an Investigational New Drug (IND) application. Many states gave up as soon as the officials in charge of the programs confronted

17. Marijuana Scheduling Petition, Denial of Petition, *Federal Register* 54, No. 249 (Dec. 29, 1988), 53784.

18. U.S. Court of Appeals, District of Columbia Circuit, Docket 90–1019, Petition for Review of Orders of the DEA, Apr. 26, 1991, 9.

19. Alabama, Alaska, Arizona, Arkansas, California, Colorado, Connecticut, Florida, Georgia, Illinois, Iowa, Louisiana, Maine, Michigan, Minnesota, Montana, Nevada, New Hampshire, New Jersey, New York, North Carolina, Ohio, Oregon, Rhode Island, South Carolina, Tennessee, Texas, Vermont, Virginia, Washington, West Virginia, and Wisconsin.

the regulatory nightmare of the relevant federal laws. Nevertheless, between 1978 and 1984, seventeen states received permission to establish programs for the use of marihuana in treating glaucoma and the nausea induced by cancer chemotherapy. Each of these programs have fallen into abeyance because of the many problems involved.

Take the case of Louisiana, where a law was passed in 1978 establishing a program that allowed a Marihuana Prescription Board to review and approve applications by physicians to treat patients with cannabis. The board would have preferred a simple procedure in which medical decisions would be entrusted to the practicing physician, but federal agencies would not supply cannabis without an IND. That would have required an enormous amount of paperwork and would have made the program intolerably cumbersome. The board therefore decided to use an already approved research program operated by the National Cancer Institute, which was limited to cancer patients and employed only synthetic THC. Marihuana itself was not made legally available to any patient in Louisiana. With these limitations, the program proved ineffective. Patients felt compelled to use illicit cannabis, and at least one was arrested.[20]

Only ten states eventually established programs in which cannabis was used as a medicine. Among these New Mexico was the first and the most successful, largely because of the efforts of a young cancer patient, Lynn Pierson. In 1978 the state legislature enacted a law allowing physicians to prescribe marihuana to patients suffering from nausea and vomiting induced by cancer chemotherapy. The law was later modified to comply with federal IND regulations requiring a research program. Considerable friction immediately developed between the FDA and the people in charge of the New Mexico program. The FDA demanded studies with placebos (inactive substances) as controls; the physicians in the New Mexico program wanted to provide sick patients with care. The FDA wanted to proceed slowly; the attitudes of the physicians reflected the urgency of their patients'

20. DEA, Marijuana Rescheduling Petition, Docket 86–22, Affidavit of Philip Jobe, Ph.D.

needs. Eventually a compromise was reached: patients would be assigned at random to treatment with marihuana cigarettes or synthetic THC capsules. But prolonged delays suggested to the New Mexico officials that the FDA was not dealing in good faith, and tensions began to grow. At one point state officials even considered using confiscated marihuana, and the chief of the State Highway Patrol was asked whether it could be supplied.

In August 1978, Lynn Pierson, who had made a heroic effort to establish a compassionate program, died of cancer without ever having received legal marihuana. Now the FDA approved the New Mexico IND, only to rescind the approval a few weeks later, after the public furor surrounding Pierson's death had faded. At that point New Mexico officials considered holding a press conference to condemn federal officials for "unethical and immoral behavior." Finally, in November 1978, the program was approved; supplies of marihuana were promised within a month, but not delivered for two months.

The random design of the program was soon violated. Patients discussed among themselves the relative merits of the two types of treatment and switched when they wanted to do so; this also gave them a sense of control over their own care. But many patients believed, despite the denials of the National Institute of Drug Abuse, that the cigarettes they received were not of adequate potency. The state never conducted an independent assay. Some patients left the program in order to buy cannabis on the streets, which they felt was better than either government marihuana or synthetic THC.

From 1978 to 1986 about 250 cancer patients in New Mexico received either marihuana or THC after conventional medications had failed to control their nausea and vomiting. For these patients both marihuana and THC were effective, but marihuana was superior. More than 90 percent reported significant or total relief from nausea and vomiting. Only three adverse effects were reported in the entire program—anxiety reactions that were easily treated by simple reassurance.[21]

21. Ibid., Affidavit of Daniel Dansak, M.D.

The successful programs in other states resembled the one in New Mexico. It was understood that "research" was merely a disguise; the aim was to relieve suffering. Although the results did not meet the methodological standards for controlled clinical research, they did confirm the effectiveness of cannabis and the advantage of smoked marihuana over oral THC. Incidentally, none of the programs reported problems with abuse or the diversion of either THC or marihuana cigarettes.

A New York State Department of Health report on the therapeutic use of cannabis asked why more patients and physicians had not enrolled in the New York program. It concluded that there were several reasons. First, physicians were skeptical because of their limited training and experience. Second, bureaucratic obstacles were enormous. As the report states, "Hospital pharmacists and administrators complain about paperwork and procedures. Physicians complain about burdensome reporting and application requirements. At least sixteen physicians have inquired into the availability of marijuana, but have chosen not to enroll in the program because they perceive a large amount of bureaucratic procedure." A third possibility was that many patients and physicians decided it was easier to get marihuana of good quality on the street.[22]

At about the same time the state programs were being instituted, growing demand forced the FDA to institute an Individual Treatment IND (commonly referred to as a Compassionate Use IND or Compassionate IND) for the use of individual physicians whose patients needed marihuana. The application process was not easy, because it was designed for an entirely different purpose—making pharmaceutical companies assure the safety of new drugs. First the patient in need of cannabis had to persuade a physician to apply to the FDA for an IND. The physician then had to file a special form with the DEA covering Schedule I drugs. If the application was approved by both agencies, the physician then had to fill out special order forms for

22. Annual Report to the Governor and Legislature on the Antonio G. Olivieri Controlled Substances Therapeutic Research Program, New York State Department of Health, Sept. 1, 1982.

marihuana, which were sent to the National Institute of Drug Abuse (NIDA). NIDA grew cannabis on a farm at the University of Mississippi—the only legal marihuana farm in the United States—and sent it to North Carolina, where it was rolled into cigarettes that were supposed to have the same potency as street marihuana (2 percent THC). NIDA then shipped the marihuana to a designated pharmacy that had to comply with stringent DEA regulations for drug security. The application process took four to eight months. Both the FDA and the DEA required constant prodding and rarely responded within the time specified by law. According to the Alliance for Cannabis Therapeutics, which helped a number of patients and physicians through the process, government agencies routinely seemed to lose some of the application forms, and the doctor had to resubmit them, sometimes more than once. Understandably, most physicians did not want to become entangled in the paperwork, especially since many also believe there is some stigma attached to prescribing cannabis.

In 1976 Robert Randall became the first patient to receive a Compassionate IND for the use of marihuana. Over the next thirteen years the government reluctantly awarded a half dozen more. Then, in 1989, the FDA was deluged with applications from people with AIDS. The case that called attention to the absurd and appalling consequences of the medical ban on marihuana was the government assault on Kenneth and Barbra Jenks, a Florida couple in their twenties who had contracted AIDS through a blood transfusion given to the husband, a hemophiliac. Both were suffering from nausea, vomiting, and appetite loss caused by AIDS or AZT; their doctor feared that Barbra Jenks would die of starvation before the disease killed her. In early 1989 the Jenkses learned about marihuana through a support group for people with AIDS. They began to smoke it and for a year they led a fairly normal life. They felt better, regained lost weight, and were able to stay out of the hospital; Kenneth Jenks even kept his full-time job.

Then someone informed on them. On March 29, 1990, ten armed narcotics officers battered down the door of their trailer home, held a gun to Barbra Jenks's head, and seized the evidence of crime, two small marihuana plants they had been growing because they could not afford to pay the street price of the drug. Cultivation of marihuana is a felony in Florida; the Jenkses faced up to five years in prison. At their trial in July they used the defense of medical necessity, which is rarely successful. The judge rejected this defense and convicted the Jenkses, although he imposed only a suspended sentence. The conviction was later overturned by a higher court and the defense of medical necessity was sustained.

The case received national publicity, and the Jenkses were able to obtain a Compassionate IND. Now the FDA was inundated with new requests from AIDS sufferers. The number of extant Compassionate INDs rose from five to thirty-four in a year. In early June 1991, Deputy National Drug Control Policy Director Herbert D. Kleber assured a national television audience that anyone with a legitimate medical need for marihuana would be able to get a Compassionate IND. But a few weeks later James O. Mason, chief of the Public Health Service, announced that the program would be suspended because it undercut the Bush administration's opposition to the use of illegal drugs. "If it is perceived that the Public Health Service is going around giving marihuana to folks, there would be a perception that this stuff can't be so bad," Mason said. He went on, "It gives a bad signal. I don't mind doing that if there is no other way of helping these people. . . . But there is not a shred of evidence that smoking marihuana assists a person with AIDS."

After keeping the program "under review" for nine months, the Public Health Service discontinued it in March 1992. Twenty-eight patients whose applications had already been approved (including some whose stories follow) were denied the promised marihuana. Thirteen patients already receiving marihuana were allowed to continue receiving it. By 1996, that number had fallen to eight. After more than twenty years in which hundreds of people have worked through state legislatures, federal courts, and administrative agencies to make marihuana available for suffering people, these eight are the only ones for whom it is not still a forbidden medicine.

2 Common Medical Uses

In the twentieth century cannabis has been proposed or shown to be useful as a medicine for many disorders and symptoms. These uses range from the proven to the speculative, but they should all be of interest to anyone concerned about human suffering. The narratives of patients illustrate most vividly not only marihuana's therapeutic properties but also the unnecessary further pain and anxiety imposed on sick people who must obtain it illegally.

CANCER CHEMOTHERAPY

Chemotherapy is one of the most important cancer treatments developed in the past several decades. Administered intravenously once every few weeks, chemotherapeutic agents are among the most powerful and toxic chemicals used in medicine. In attacking cancer cells, they also kill healthy body cells, producing extremely unpleasant and dangerous side effects. Among the most widely used chemotherapeutic agents are cisplatin (Platinol), doxorubicin (Adriamycin), cyclophosphamide (Cytoxan), ifosfamide (Ifex), and nitrogen mustard derivatives, including such drugs as melphalan (Alkeran) and chlorambucil (Leukeran).

Cisplatin can cause deafness or life-threatening kidney failure. Ifosfamide can cause bleeding and bruising; cyclophosphamide suppresses the immune system; doxorubicin can destroy heart muscle. Nitrogen mustard derivatives are so toxic that they eat away the skin or any other tissue they touch. If the intravenous needle through which they are being delivered leaks or slips out of the vein, the resulting scar tissue may cause the patient to lose the use of an arm. Most of these drugs also cause hair loss, and any of them may cause a second type of cancer while suppressing the original disease. Doses must be carefully calculated to prevent kidney, heart, or respiratory failure.

But the most common and for many patients the most troublesome side effect of these drugs is profound nausea and vomiting. Retching (dry heaves) may last for hours or even days after each treatment, followed by days and even weeks of nausea. Patients may break bones or rupture the esophagus while vomiting. The sense of loss of control can be emotionally devastating. Furthermore, many patients eat almost nothing because they cannot stand the sight or smell of food. As they lose weight and strength, they find it more and more difficult to sustain the will to live.

Patients become more apprehensive with each successive treatment. Some develop a conditioned reaction that causes them to vomit when they walk into the treatment room or even before they arrive at the hospital. A few have been known to vomit reflexively on seeing a member of the treatment team on the street. If the nausea and vomiting cannot be controlled, the patient's complaints may cause doctors to lower the dose and jeopardize the effectiveness of the therapy. For many patients, the side effects of chemotherapy seem worse than the cancer itself, and they discontinue treatment, not only to eliminate the discomfort, but also to regain control over their lives. Some insist on stopping even though they know it means certain death. In otherwise treatable patients who refuse therapy, the nausea and vomiting should be considered a potentially lethal form of toxicity.

Many patients, fortunately, get sufficient relief from such standard antiemetic drugs as prochlorperazine (Compazine) or the newer ondansetron (Zofran) and granisetron (Kytril). But in some cases these drugs never work or soon stop working. Zofran is now considered the most effective of the standard antiemetics, but often it must be administered over a period of hours through an intravenous drip while the patient remains in a hospital bed, at a cost of hundreds of dollars per treatment.

As the results of various state research programs indicate, marihuana may be a remarkably effective substitute for standard drugs. In one study of fifty-six patients who got no relief from standard antiemetic agents, 78 percent became symptom-free when they smoked marihuana.[1] One of us (L.G.) has had a personal encounter with this therapeutic effect:

Early in 1972, after the death of Sidney Farber, the Harvard children's oncologist for whom the Sidney Farber Cancer Research Center was named, my wife and I were invited to dinner at the home of a fellow Harvard Medical School faculty member. He wanted me to meet Emil Frei, who had arrived from Houston to serve as Dr. Farber's successor.

At dinner, Dr. Frei told me about an eighteen-year-old Houston man with leukemia who had become more and more resistant to cancer chemotherapy because he could no longer tolerate the nausea and vomiting. His doctors and his family were finding it increasingly difficult to persuade him to take the drug on which his life depended.

One day, to Dr. Frei's surprise, the young man willingly agreed to take the drug and from then on offered no resistance to chemotherapy. He eventually revealed that he had been smoking marihuana twenty minutes before each session; it prevented all vomiting and even the slightest hint of nausea. Dr. Frei asked me whether this property was mentioned in the nineteenth-century medical literature on cannabis, and I told him that it was. On the way home my wife, Betsy, who had listened with great interest, suggested that we obtain some cannabis for our son Danny.

1. V. Vinciguerra, T. Moore, and E. Brennan, "Inhalation Marihuana as an Antiemetic for Cancer Chemotherapy," *New York State Journal of Medicine* 88 (October 1988): 525–527.

Danny was first given the diagnosis of acute lymphatic leukemia in July 1967; he was ten years old. For the first few years he was good-natured about his treatment at Children's Hospital in Boston and even about the occasional need for hospitalization. But in 1971 he started taking the first of the drugs that cause severe nausea and vomiting.

Danny was one of those patients in whom these reactions were uncontrollable and not sufficiently alleviated by standard antiemetics. He would start to vomit shortly after treatment and continue retching for up to eight hours. He vomited in the car as we drove home, and on arriving he had to lie in bed with his head over a bucket on the floor. Still, I was shocked when Betsy suggested that we find cannabis for Danny. I objected because it was against the law and because it might embarrass staff members at the hospital, who had been so remarkable in their commitment to Danny's care. I dismissed the idea.

Danny's next treatment was two weeks later. When I arrived, Betsy and Danny were already in the treatment room. I shall never forget my surprise. Normally my wife and son were in a state of great anxiety before the treatment began, but this time they were completely relaxed, and, what is more, seemed almost to be playing a joke on me.

Finally, they let me in on the secret. On the way to the clinic that morning they had stopped near Wellesley High School, and Betsy had asked one of Danny's friends to get her some marihuana. Once he recovered from his disbelief, the friend had run off and reappeared a few minutes later with a small amount of marihuana. Betsy and Danny had smoked it in the parking lot of the hospital just before entering the clinic.

My surprise gave way to relief as I saw how comfortable Danny was. He did not protest as he was given the medicine, and we were all delighted when no nausea or vomiting followed. On the way home he asked his mother if he could stop for a submarine sandwich, and when he got home he began his usual activities instead of going straight to bed. We could scarcely believe it.

The next day I called Dr. Norman Jaffe, the physician who was in charge of Danny's care. I explained what had happened and said that while I did not want to embarrass him or the rest of the medical staff, I could not forbid Danny to smoke marihuana before his next treatment. Dr. Jaffe responded by suggesting that Danny smoke marihuana in his presence in the treatment room.

Danny did that the next time. When he was given the chemotherapeutic agent, Dr. Jaffe could observe for himself that he was completely relaxed. Afterward he again asked for a submarine sandwich. From then on he used marihuana before every treatment, and we were all much more comfortable during the remaining year of his life.

Doctor Jaffe asked me to join him in reporting our observations to Dr. Frei, who was sufficiently interested to perform the first clinical experiment on the use of cannabis in cancer chemotherapy.[2]

Cannabis has been investigated as a medicine even more rarely in children than in adults. Frei and his colleagues wanted to study the use of smoked cannabis in children with cancer, but the FDA permitted them to give only delta-9-THC to adults. Israeli researchers have recently found that another cannabinoid, delta-8-THC (a congener of delta-9-THC with less psychoactive potency) effectively prevented nausea and vomiting in eight children aged three to fifteen suffering from various hematologic (blood) cancers. During treatment for up to eight months with a variety of chemotherapeutic drugs, delta-8-THC was completely effective with negligible side effects.[3]

Arnold and Mae Nutt, now in their late seventies, raised three sons in Beaverton, Michigan. In 1963, shortly after his fifth birthday, Dana, the middle child, was found to have bone cancer. After surgery he re-

2. S. E. Sallan, N. E. Zinberg, and E. Frei, III, "Antiemetic Effect of Delta-9-tetrahydrocannabinol in Patients Receiving Cancer Chemotherapy," *New England Journal of Medicine* 293 (1975): 795–797.

3. A. Abrahamov and R. Mechoulam, "An Efficient New Cannabinoid Antiemetic in Pediatric Oncology," *Life Sciences* 56:23–24 (May 5, 1995): 2097–2102.

ceived chemotherapy and radiation treatments for three months. The treatments made him very ill but did not halt the spread of the cancer, and he died in 1967. For years the Nutts struggled to recover from their grief and the financial burden imposed by their son's illness. Then, in 1978, their oldest son, Keith, developed testicular cancer at the age of twenty-two. Mae Nutt tells his story:

Surgeons operated on Keith, removing the diseased testicle and a large number of lymph nodes. They believed they had cut out all of the cancer. Keith made a determined effort to remain active. He resumed working, and all appeared to be going well, but nine months later he discovered that his other testicle was hard and enlarged. Surgeons immediately removed it, and he was told that he would require extensive chemotherapy as well. He was given cisplatin, a new, highly toxic drug that made him extremely ill. He would vomit violently for eight to ten hours, and afterward was so profoundly nauseated that he could not bear to look at or smell food. Compazine and other antiemetic drugs provided no noticeable relief.

In less than two months our son lost at least thirty pounds. He began to vomit bile. When there was nothing to vomit, he would simply retch and convulse. It was horrible for us to watch our child suffer such anguish from the disease and the treatment. At one point Keith told me he did not want to become like his deceased brother Dana—so sick he could not take care of himself, completely incapacitated, and a burden on the rest of the family. He told me that when things got that bad, he wanted to be able to kill himself. He made me promise that when there was no hope, I would help him end his life.

One evening I read a newspaper article about a cancer patient who had received a brown bag of marihuana on his doorstep. The article noted that medical evidence suggested it could reduce the severe nausea and vomiting caused by many anticancer therapies. The idea that marihuana had medical uses was new to my husband and me. At first I laughed at the story. It seemed unlikely that marihuana would just suddenly appear on someone's doorstep.

As a parent I was strongly opposed to marihuana and other illegal drugs. My husband and I made sure our sons knew exactly how we felt. We do not doubt that they may have experimented with marihuana while growing up, but we are also sure they had no drug problems and no illusions about our stern opposition to drug use. It was hard to believe that an illegal drug could be of any help. If marihuana had medical value, we thought that the government would know and would make it legally available by prescription.

But we were desperate, so we told Keith what we had read. He replied that other patients in the hospital who were receiving chemotherapy smoked marihuana to reduce the side effects and said it worked. We proceeded to contact our state representative, Robert Young, and asked him whether we could legally obtain marihuana for Keith. We were surprised to learn that a bill to legalize marihuana for the treatment of glaucoma and cancer was scheduled to come before the Michigan legislature. Representative Young also put us in touch with Mr. Roger Winthrop, a man who was working on the legislation with representatives and senators. He provided information on the medical uses of marihuana and told us that physicians and patients in several states had already succeeded in getting them to pass laws making it available to seriously ill patients like Keith.

Shortly after my husband and I read these materials, Keith had another round of chemotherapy, and, as always, it made him dreadfully sick. We could not stand by and watch him suffer, but, as an older couple, we did not have the slightest idea where to find marihuana. In desperation we asked a close friend for help, an ordained Presbyterian minister who worked with local youth groups. Several days later he appeared at our door with some marihuana. It was the first time we had ever seen any.

The next day we took the marihuana to Keith in the hospital. After he smoked it his vomiting abruptly stopped. The sudden change was amazing to see. Marihuana also put an end to his nausea. When he smoked it he was constantly hungry and actually began to put on weight. His mental outlook also underwent a startling improvement. Before he started to smoke marihuana Keith would come home from chemotherapy, shut himself in his bedroom, stuff towels under the door to keep out the smell of dinner cooking, and remain in his room or the bathroom vomiting all evening. The cancer and chemotherapy made him act like a wounded animal, timid and retiring. He had intense hot and cold flashes. His joints became swollen and painful. His hair fell out and he felt sick all over. Large pieces of skin came off at the place where the injections were given.

Smoking marihuana dramatically changed his life. Immediately before the chemotherapy he smoked one marihuana cigarette, and afterward, if he felt queasy, all or part of a second. When we arrived home he stayed in the living room and talked with his brother and father. He joined the family for dinner and ate more than his share. He became outgoing and talkative, part of our family again. He never once experienced an adverse effect. Marihuana was the safest, most benign drug he received in the course of his battle against cancer.

We made certain that all of his doctors and nurses were aware of the situation; none objected and some clearly approved. We even arranged for him to smoke marihuana in his hospital room. In effect, reasonable people caring for Keith decided that the law did not match the reality of his needs.

We learned that many cancer patients were smoking marihuana and most told their doctors, who approved but were not willing to say in public what they told their patients in their offices.

My husband and I came to resent the fact that Keith's therapy was illegal. We felt like criminals. We are honest, simple people and hate having to sneak around. We were uncomfortable asking our closest friends, our minister, and our other son, Marc, to risk arrest in order to provide Keith with the medicine he so obviously needed. We were also concerned about other parents who might not know that marihuana could help end their child's misery. We asked Keith whether we could tell his story to a local newspaper, the *Bay City Times*, to help other cancer patients. He agreed on the condition that we not supply details about the nature of his cancer and the surgical removal of his testes. As a young man in his twenties, he wanted at least that much of his life to remain private.

On the day the article about Keith appeared in the newspaper, we went to Lansing to testify before the Michigan Senate Judiciary Committee on the medical marihuana legislation. The hearings generated considerable publicity, and we began to receive phone calls from other cancer patients in Michigan and throughout the United States. Keith often spoke with them late into the night. Cancer patients and their relatives asked him for help and advice on how to smoke properly, how much to use, and how often. He even went on "house calls" several times to show patients how to roll the cigarettes or inhale the smoke. This opportunity to help others gave Keith great joy.

One day shortly after the hearings we found a small brown bag of marihuana in our mailbox. There was no note, no identification, just an ounce of marihuana. I remembered the newspaper story I had laughed at, the one in which marihuana appeared on someone's doorstep. Soon we received more marihuana in the mail. The donors usually remained anonymous, but not always. An Episcopal priest, for example, brought marihuana to our house and said he thought we would know who might benefit from it. As news spread through the grapevine, we heard from some familiar folks. One day we received a call from a woman who had attended elementary school with Arnold, my husband. She invited us to her home and offered us a cigar box filled with marihuana. She explained that her husband, recently deceased, had smoked it to help control terminal cancer pain. She had no use for it now but did not want to throw it away.

When my husband and I returned to Lansing for additional

legislative hearings, Keith was back in the hospital and his cancer was spreading again. This time we were joined by another family, the Negens, of Grand Rapids, who had testified at the previous hearing without giving their names. Their daughter Deborah, twenty-one, was receiving chemotherapy for leukemia, and marihuana was the only drug that relieved the debilitating side effects. The Reverend Negen is pastor of the very conservative Dutch Christian Reform Church in Grand Rapids. He testified that he had prayed for guidance and realized that if using marihuana to help his daughter offended his congregation, he would have to leave his church. He spoke movingly about having to send his own young sons into the streets of Grand Rapids to buy marihuana for his daughter. It was easy for us to understand Reverend Negen's distress. Like us, he was being forced to break the law to provide for his child's medical needs.

Deborah Negen herself was even more eloquent and moving as she pleaded with the committee to consider that other seriously ill people were suffering needlessly.

On October 10, 1979, the Michigan House voted 100 to 0 in favor of making marihuana available to patients like Keith. On October 15, the Senate concurred, 33 to 1. On the evening of Sunday, October 21, my husband and I told Keith that the Michigan Marihuana as Medicine bill would be signed into law the next day. Keith was happy that his efforts had made a difference. He smiled and said good night. Early in the next morning he died, and later that day the bill was signed into law.

Six months after they were married in 1969, Mona Taft's husband, Harris, noticed a lump on his neck. A biopsy performed at the Massachusetts General Hospital in Boston revealed Hodgkin's disease, a malignancy of the lymph nodes. Mona Taft tells their story:

At the time of diagnosis Harris was gravely ill, but not yet showing the advanced, manifest symptoms of Hodgkin's disease. He immediately underwent the first of many surgical procedures: his spleen and affected lymph glands were removed through an incision that ran from his pelvic bone to his chest. As soon as the wound healed and he recovered some of his strength, he began to receive the first in what was to be a decade of anticancer treatments.

Despite doctors' warnings, we were totally unprepared for the devastating effects of chemotherapy. Within ninety minutes after receiving his first chemotherapy treatment, my husband began to vomit, and the vomiting persisted for endless hours. When there was nothing left to throw up, he would get the dry heaves. A day later the vomiting would subside, but he remained so nauseated that he could not eat or even stand the sight or smell of food. The doctors prescribed a series of antiemetic drugs like Compazine. None of them worked. Harris received chemotherapy at least once a month for nearly a year. It seemed to help suppress his cancer, but it also took a terrible toll on the quality of his life.

In the next seven years Harris was in and out of remission several times. Each time the cancer returned, it was more widespread, the drugs used to fight it were more toxic, and the adverse reactions became more severe. Meanwhile Harris underwent many more surgical procedures, including the removal of cancerous tissue that had spread to his brain. Later he began to find walking difficult because of cancerous tissue in his spine that was pinching the nerves leading to his legs. These tumors, too, were surgically removed. As the disease continued to spread, Harris underwent exploratory abdominal surgery; the doctors found too much cancer to remove. More chemotherapy was recommended, and radiation treatments were added, causing further nausea. Each day was becoming more and more painful for him.

One day in 1977, when we arrived at the treatment room where Harris was to receive the injection, he bolted and ran down the corridor. I found him a bit later, wandering the halls. He told me he couldn't take any more chemotherapy. He was at wit's end, exhausted by the disease, terrified by the effects of the drugs that were supposed to prolong his life. I have never before or since seen a man so genuinely and deeply frightened. Harris had come to fear the treatments more than the cancer and, he admitted, more than death itself. He told me he would choose dying over further chemotherapy.

One of the nurse practitioners overheard us and interrupted; she said she understood our problem and suggested that Harris smoke marihuana to relieve the nausea and vomiting. We were startled. Although Harris had occasionally smoked marihuana socially, he couldn't believe it would help. We asked Harris's doctor about marihuana, and he said that he couldn't encourage us to do anything illegal, but many of his younger patients were smoking marihuana and it seemed to reduce their trouble with nausea and vomiting. The message was pretty clear: Try marihuana and see if it helps. Harris had a strong will to live and, as he said, nothing to lose, so he decided to give chemotherapy one more chance and smoke some marihuana beforehand. I did not have much hope.

When Harris went for his next chemotherapy session, he was so frightened he forgot to bring his marihuana; I had to take it to him after he called from his hospital room. Doctors, nurses, and orderlies must have seen him smoking it, but no one said anything. It was as if we had all reached an unspoken understanding. After the chemotherapy I decided to stay with Harris through the night in case he needed my help. But this time there was no vomiting; he slept like a baby. It was his first full night of restful sleep in nearly seven years of anticancer treatments. The next morning he actually ate breakfast, a real breakthrough. No vomiting. No nausea. And he actually wanted to eat! I cannot describe how relieved and excited we were. Why hadn't someone told us sooner? Why had my husband gone through all those years of needless suffering?

Usually Harris was sick for weeks after receiving chemotherapy; this time he was ready to go back to work in forty-eight hours. From that time on he smoked marihuana whenever he had chemotherapy. The results were dramatic. He started to regain lost weight, and his mood improved remarkably. He became more active and outgoing, and we began to do things together that I thought we would never be able to do again. It was clear that his doctors knew what he was doing and approved; they couldn't help noticing the sudden improvement in his condition.

It is impossible for me to adequately describe what a profound difference marihuana made. Before using marihuana Harris felt ill all the time, could not eat, could not even stand the smell of food cooking. Afterward, he remained active, ate regular meals, and could be himself. His mood, his manner, and his overall outlook were transformed. And of course, marihuana prolonged his life by allowing him to continue chemotherapy. In two years of smoking it, he never had an adverse or untoward reaction. Marihuana was the least dangerous drug my husband received during the nine years he was treated for cancer.

During this period (1977–1979) Harris and I learned that many other cancer patients were smoking marihuana for the same purpose. Most of them had learned about it from their doctors, who could only offer hints and suggestions and rarely discussed the subject openly and thoroughly. They could not legally prescribe the drug to them or supervise their use of it, yet they could prescribe highly toxic chemotherapeutic drugs, dangerously addictive narcotics, and radiation treatments. I remember thinking how crazy it was.

Since Harris's death in 1979, I have had time to reflect on the meanness of a law that deprived him of his legal right to obtain the one drug that actually relieved his nausea and vomiting. I become upset, then enraged when I realize that other cancer patients are being denied such relief. I think about older people who might not know where to find marihuana or might be too frightened to smoke an illegal drug without close medical supervision. And I think about children and teenagers whose parents must face an agonizing choice between breaking the law and watching as their child suffers.

At the age of thirty-seven, Richard Brookhiser, a senior editor of the *National Review* and a columnist for the *New York Observer,* developed testicular cancer:

> In the spring of 1992, I made the unwelcome discovery that I had testicular cancer. The treatment for this ailment is straightforward: cisplatin, one of the stronger chemicals used in chemotherapy (I came to think of it as the Chemo of Champions). But any chemotherapy is poison, killing millions of cells in order to kill the thousands that matter.
>
> I took four courses of cisplatin—once a month, for five days at a time. Zofran [ondansetron], a powerful antinausea drug, had just been introduced, and I also did mental imaging to make the chemotherapy more tolerable (visualized the cisplatin as raucous Jamaican street-sweepers). But as the second course of chemotherapy ended, I could feel that I would need extra help holding the nausea at bay, and so I turned to pot.
>
> I had smoked marihuana maybe a dozen times in college, and the experience was mixed. My experience of pot-heads was unmixed: I found them boring and silly (I still do). But I knew that it made one hungry, and that this was the effect I would be relying on now.
>
> None of my doctors at New York University Medical Center, where I was treated, or at Memorial Sloan-Kettering Cancer Center, where I went for a consultation, discouraged me from using marihuana. But they of course could not prescribe it. They might have prescribed Marinol, the pill form of THC, but a pill did not seem like a terribly useful way to fight nausea. So my wife and I had to break the law. We even went to an East Village paraphernalia shop and found, among the heavy metal T-shirts and the stashes designed to look like beer cans, a wooden one-hitter. This seemed to be on the near side of legality, though the police closed the shop a few months later.
>
> The harbinger of nausea, like clouds coming in before a storm, is a several-minute-long period of heaviness and unease. During

my third course of chemotherapy, whenever I felt the warning signs, I would go to the bathroom in my hospital room and light up. As a result, my third helping of cisplatin was nausea-free. By the fourth, even marihuana couldn't do the whole job. But I think it is reasonable to assume that without it I would have had a harder time.

My experience of cancer was short—the four courses of chemotherapy cured me—and given the high success rate of cisplatin with testicular cancer (over 90 percent), I was never in serious danger. But my near-death experience was enough to show me the importance for cancer patients of maintaining morale, while my near-vomit experience demonstrated the discouraging effects of nausea. Nothing is more depressing than kneeling on a hospital bathroom floor, staring at the American Standard logo.

One surprising effect of my marihuana use is that I have become the perfect citizen of a drug-free America. Anyone who fears that the use of medical marihuana will cause an upsurge in recreational use should fear not. Only someone who was already an aficionado could tolerate even looking at a joint again after passing through the hospital experience. Yet if I or anyone I love should ever be in a similar situation, I would not hesitate to turn to pot again.

If the federal government does not change the law in the interim, I would have to become a criminal again. It is outrageous that a helpful, harmless drug cannot be prescribed by doctors or bought over the counter like aspirin. It is also sobering to reflect that, as a member of the media elite, living in liberal Manhattan, I was at minimal risk of punishment. But wherever prosecutors have less to do, an average person runs a risk indeed if he seeks to help himself with medical marihuana.

I see no conflict between these convictions and my principles, which are those of a conservative Republican. Conservatives dislike bureaucracies run amok, and the bureaucracy which forbids the medical use of marihuana is a classic example. Conservatives resist magical thinking—the notion that bad *things* cause bad deeds—when liberals apply it to firearms: the same principle should apply to drugs.

I find substantial private agreement when I mention these points to fellow conservatives. I hope future Republican Congresses and White Houses will see that medical marihuana is a freedom issue, too.

Brookhiser's wife, Jeanne Safer, a psychologist who has treated many people for problems of substance abuse in her psychotherapeutic practice, supplied her own perspective on Richard's experience:

Four years ago, my husband, Richard Brookhiser, was diagnosed with testicular cancer. The chemotherapy regime which saved his life included cisplatin, a drug notorious for the nausea it induces. Even though the new and potent antiemetic medication Zofran was prescribed to counteract this side effect, we were advised by several friends who had themselves been through the treatment that smoking marihuana was more effective, particularly for younger people.

As Rick has written, Zofran held his nausea at bay into his second of four rounds of treatment. When it became clear to me that it would no longer suffice, I bought marihuana for him. Smoking it as needed permitted him to eat, to think, to work, and to feel a modicum of control over his body and his life throughout this ordeal.

I consider myself fortunate to have been able to obtain pot so easily and painlessly; a friend delivered it on rollerblades to my door within the hour, and several others offered to provide high-quality reinforcements as needed. What, I wondered, would I have done had I lived elsewhere, not had the money, or not known where to go?

I frequently treat drug abusers in my practice and am opposed to virtually all drug use. However, I see no relation whatsoever between the misuse of marihuana by the healthy and the therapeutic use of it by the sick.

As a clinical psychologist, I was struck by several important

functions of marihuana in easing chemotherapy. Marihuana relieved both of us: physiologically, it allowed Rick to endure most
of his treatment with his nausea considerably diminished, and
psychologically, it gave me something active and positive I could
do for him. There are few things as difficult as watching someone
you love suffer as you stand helplessly by. For patients themselves, knowing that relief is available, effective, and—more important—under their own control can lessen the dread and make
the suffering more tolerable. Smoking pot allows a person to titrate the dosage and thus treats anticipatory anxiety as well as
nausea. I would use marihuana myself for this purpose and recommend it to patients, colleagues, and friends.

To deny this assistance to anyone who needs it is unconscionable. It is bad medicine and worse psychology.

Here is another testimony to the powers of cannabis as an antiemetic, from Stephen Jay Gould, Alexander Professor of Geology at
Harvard University and the author of many highly regarded books
and essays on biological evolution:

> I am a member of a very small, very fortunate, and very select
> group—the first survivors of the previously incurable cancer, ab-
> dominal mesothelioma. Our treatment involved a carefully bal-
> anced mixture of all three standard modalities—surgery, radi-
> ation, and chemotherapy. Not pleasant, to be sure, but consider
> the alternative.
>
> Any cancer survivor of such intensive treatment—indeed, any-
> one who has endured aggressive medical battles against any dis-
> ease—knows firsthand the enormous importance of the "psycho-
> logical factor." Now I am an old-fashioned rationalist of the most
> unreconstructed sort. I brook no mysticism, no romantic South-
> ern California nonsense, about the power of mind and spirit. I
> assume that positive attitudes and optimism have salutary effects
> because mental states can feed back upon the body through the
> immune system. In any case, I think that everyone would grant
> an important role to the maintenance of spirit through adversity;

when the mind gives up, the body too often follows. (And if cure is not the ultimate outcome, quality of remaining life becomes, if anything, even more important.)

Nothing is more discouraging, more destructive of the possibility of such a positive attitude—and I do speak from personal experience here—than the serious side effects induced by so many treatments. Radiation and chemotherapy are often accompanied by long periods of intense and uncontrollable nausea. The mind begins to associate the agent of potential cure with the very worst aspect of the disease—for the pain and suffering of the side effects is often worse than the distress induced by the tumor itself. Once this happens, the possibility for an essential psychological boost and comfort may disappear—for the treatment seems worse than the disease itself. In other words, I am trying to say that the control of severe and long-lasting side effects in cancer treatment is not merely a question of comfort (though Lord only knows that comfort to the suffering is enough of a rationale), but an absolutely essential ingredient in the possibility of cure.

I had surgery, followed by a month of radiation, chemotherapy, more surgery, and a subsequent year of additional chemotherapy. I found that I could control the less severe nausea of radiation by conventional medicines. But when I started intravenous chemotherapy (Adriamycin), absolutely nothing in the available arsenal of antiemetics worked at all. I was miserable and came to dread the frequent treatments with an almost perverse intensity.

I had heard that marihuana often worked well against nausea. I was reluctant to try it because I have never smoked any substance habitually (and didn't even know how to inhale). Moreover, I had tried marihuana twice (in the usual context of growing up in the sixties) and had hated it. (I am something of a Puritan on the subject of substances that, in any way, dull or alter mental states—for I value my rational mind with an academician's overweening arrogance. I do not drink alcohol at all, and have never used drugs in any "recreational" sense.) But anything to avoid nausea and the perverse wish it induces for an end of treatment.

The rest of the story is short and sweet. Marihuana worked like a charm. I disliked the "side effect" of mental blurring (the "main effect" for recreational users), but the sheer bliss of not experiencing nausea—and then not having to fear it for all the days intervening between treatments—was the greatest boost I received in all my year of treatment, and surely had a most important effect upon my eventual cure. It is beyond my comprehension—and I fancy I am able to comprehend a lot, including much nonsense—that any humane person would withhold such a beneficial substance from people in such great need simply because others use it for different purposes.

A major advantage of cannabis as an aid in cancer chemotherapy is its relatively low cost. Even with the present "prohibition tariff" it is far less expensive than most of the conventional medicines it would replace, as this account by Paul Kuhn, a businessman, indicates:

My wife and I discovered the benefits of marihuana during her treatments for advanced breast cancer. The first regimen she underwent consisted of four treatments with three anticancer agents. The treatments took place two weeks apart and lasted one day each. Each began with an IV drip of methotrexate in the oncologist's office. Then she went home wearing a small pump activated by body heat that infused Adriamycin (doxorubicin) for twenty-four hours. The next day she returned to her oncologist to have the pump removed and received a shot of fluorouracil.

To prevent nausea she smoked marihuana, and it worked perfectly. A single puff brought immediate relief. She was never sick and continued to eat well. Although her oncologists could not prescribe marihuana, they supported her decision to smoke and made their offices available for the purpose. During one treatment she needed a blood transfusion in the hospital cancer center, so she brought along her pipe. A nurse asked the center's supervisor for permission and was told that the hospital's legal counsel had determined that smoking marihuana "is in the patient's best interest."

A few weeks after this introductory round of treatments, tests were run to see whether the tumor had responded. It had, so the second regimen began: high-dose chemotherapy followed by a stem-cell transplant. This was recommended by our oncologists as the only hope for a durable remission. Stem cells are the young cells in bone marrow that mature into the various types of blood cell. The high-dose chemotherapy that kills breast cancer also kills stem cells, but if they are harvested before chemotherapy and returned afterward, bone marrow can be revived and the patient can recover from an otherwise fatal megadose of anticancer drugs.

Knowing that the nausea would be worse this time, my wife consulted her oncologists, her brother (a physician), and nurses with experience in treating cancer patients in her circumstances. She decided to use marihuana again, and again it worked beautifully.

During the course of her treatment my wife consumed less than $200 worth of cannabis. The necessary dose of Zofran (ondansetron), the antiemetic our oncologist first recommended, would have cost one hundred times that amount. Not that cost was a factor in her choice of treatments. She simply decided that marihuana was more likely to be effective and less likely to have serious side effects. In fact, she did take Zofran intravenously once when she forgot her marihuana pipe, and the cost was $600. A friend whose wife had the same treatment says the total cost of Zofran and its administration was more than $20,000.

Obviously, Zofran produces substantial revenue for its manufacturer and for those who dispense it. I thought of this when I learned that the Partnership for a Drug-Free America opposes allowing physicians to prescribe marihuana. The Partnership is headed by James Burke, the former president of Johnson & Johnson, and its sponsors include major pharmaceutical companies (as well as the principal distributors of alcohol and tobacco). No doubt Mr. Burke is a man of integrity and the Partnership's corporate donors have a sincere interest in curbing drug abuse. But it is unseemly (and a terrible conflict of interest) for drug companies to advocate the arrest of physicians and patients who get relief from marihuana.

Some of the other patients whose cases we discuss seem to differ with Kuhn about the price of marihuana, but the differences are easy to reconcile. The prohibition tariff makes the street price much higher than necessary, but even at that inflated price it is often less expensive than other available medications.

Since 1985 oncologists have been legally permitted to administer a synthetic THC, dronabinol (the common brand name is Marinol) orally in capsule form, and almost 100,000 doses were prescribed in 1989. But inhaled cannabis may be preferable for several reasons. For one thing, oral THC is subject to the vagaries of bioavailability. This means that two patients who take the same amount may absorb different proportions of the dose, and a given patient may respond differently on different days, depending on the condition of the intestinal tract and other factors. Furthermore, the effects of smoked cannabis are perceived almost immediately, so patients can smoke slowly and take only what they need for a therapeutic effect. Patients who swallow dronabinol may discover after an hour or so that they have taken too much for comfort or not enough to relieve their symptoms. In any case, a patient who is severely nauseated and constantly vomiting may find it almost impossible to keep the capsule down.[4]

In 1979 Alfred Chang of the National Cancer Institute studied fifteen patients with bone cancer, comparing the antiemetic effects of oral and smoked delta-9-THC with corresponding placebos.[5] The

4. Because of the difficulties with oral administration of THC, there has been some interest in developing a suppository. See M. A. ElSohly, D. F. Stanford, E. C. Harland, A. H. Hikal, L. A. Walker, T. L. Little, Jr., J. N. Rider, and A. B. Jones, "Rectal Bioavailability of Delta-9-tetrahydrocannabinol from the Hemisuccinate Ester in Monkeys," *Journal of Pharmaceutical Sciences* 80 (October 1991): 924–945.

5. The THC was suspended in sesame oil and placed in gelatin capsules; seemingly identical placebo capsules contained only sesame oil. The placebo cigarettes contained marihuana from which the cannabinoids had been extracted; the active cigarettes were prepared from these placebo cigarettes by injecting THC through a needle.

patients served as their own controls. THC was clearly effective in reducing nausea and vomiting. Seventy-two percent of the patients were nauseated and vomiting while taking a placebo. When the concentration of THC in their blood was low, 44 percent suffered from nausea and vomiting; at moderate concentrations, only 21 percent were nauseated and vomited; at fairly high concentrations just 6 percent did. Thus the effectiveness of THC depended on how much was absorbed into the bloodstream, and the investigators were able to show that smoked THC was absorbed more reliably.[6]

Furthermore, dronabinol makes some patients anxious and uncomfortable—especially older people who have had no previous experience with cannabis. One reason is the difficulty of titrating the dose of oral THC to control the amount that reaches the blood and brain. Another possibility, suggested by the work of Peruvian researchers, is that cannabidiol, one of the many substances in marihuana smoke, reduces anxiety provoked by delta-9-THC.[7] Thus, smoked marihuana may be both more effective and more comfortable to use than oral THC. We have already noted that patients in the state programs of the early 1980s almost universally preferred it.

Marihuana taken in a drink or in food shares with dronabinol the disadvantages of delayed onset, long-lasting effects and difficulty in titrating the dose, but it is probably less likely to generate anxiety because it contains cannabidiol. Experienced users, in any case, rarely suffer discomfort from cannabis, so that is unlikely to be a problem for a patient who uses it regularly. The main risk of whole cannabis taken by mouth is undermedication rather than overmedication. Nineteenth-century physicians, when they prescribed oral *Cannabis indica* preparations such as Tilden's solution, knew that cannabis was remarkably safe but also knew about the imprecision of dosage and

6. A. E. Chang, et al., "Delta-9-tetrahydrocannabinol as an Antiemetic in Cancer Patients Receiving High-dose Methotrexate: A Prospective, Randomized Evaluation," *Annals of Internal Medicine* 91 (1979): 819–824.

7. A. W. Zuardi, I. Shirakawa, E. Finkelbarb, and I. G. Karniol, "Action of Cannabidiol on the Anxiety and Other Effects Produced by Delta-9-THC in Normal Subjects," *Psychopharmacology* 76 (1976): 245–250.

variability of absorption. Therefore they preferred to err on the side of giving more rather than less.

In the spring of 1990 two investigators randomly selected more than two thousand members of the American Society of Clinical Oncology (one-third of the total membership) and mailed them an anonymous questionnaire to learn their views on the use of cannabis in cancer chemotherapy. Almost half of the recipients responded. Although the investigators acknowledge that this group was self-selected and that there might be a response bias, their results provide a rough estimate of the views of specialists on the use of Marinol and smoked marihuana.

Only 43 percent said the available legal antiemetic drugs (including oral synthetic THC) provided adequate relief to all or most of their patients, and less than 46 percent said the side effects of these drugs were a serious problem for only a few. Forty-four percent had recommended the illegal use of marihuana to at least one patient, and half would prescribe it to some patients if it were legal. On the average they considered smoked marihuana more effective than oral synthetic THC and roughly as safe.[8] Since this survey was conducted, many more oncologists presumably have learned about the value of cannabis.

GLAUCOMA

Glaucoma is a disorder that results from an imbalance of pressure within the eye. The eyeball must be almost perfectly spherical to focus light accurately on the retina. Its shape is maintained by the pressure of an internal fluid, the aqueous humor. If the eye produces too much of this fluid or the channels through which it flows out are blocked, the increasing pressure may damage the optic nerve, which carries impulses from the eye to the brain. Glaucoma afflicts 1.5 percent of the population at age fifty and about 5 percent at age seventy.

8. R. Doblin and M. A. R. Kleiman, "Marihuana as Antiemetic Medicine: A Survey of Oncologists' Attitudes and Experiences," *Journal of Clinical Oncology* 9 (1991): 1314–1319.

Almost one million Americans suffer from the disorder, and every year 80,000 are blinded by it. That makes glaucoma the second leading cause of blindness in the United States (after degeneration of the retina in old age), accounting for 10 percent of adult-onset cases. Most glaucoma is of the open-angle or chronic simple type, in which the channels narrow gradually and the pressure within rises slowly. The resulting loss of peripheral vision may go unnoticed until the disease is well advanced. Early detection and careful monitoring and control of intraocular pressure are necessary to avoid irreversible damage.

Today glaucoma is treated chiefly with eyedrops containing beta-blockers such as timolol (Timoptic), which inhibit the activity of epinephrine (adrenaline). They are highly effective but may have serious side effects; they may induce depression, aggravate asthma, slow the heart rate, and increase the risk of heart failure. Paradoxically, epinephrine-like eyedrops can also be effective in treating glaucoma, but they may irritate the white of the eye and aggravate hypertension and heart disease. Miotics (drugs that contract the pupil), such as pilocarpine, are also prescribed for glaucoma, although less often now than in the past. They are generally safe for the heart, respiratory, and digestive systems but can cause blurred vision, impaired night vision, and cataracts. Patients may also be given pills containing a carbonic anhydrase inhibitor, which reduces the production of aqueous humor. Carbonic anhydrase inhibitors may cause loss of appetite, nausea, diarrhea, headaches, numbness and tingling, depression and fatigue, kidney stones, and, rarely, a fatal blood disorder. Fifty percent of glaucoma patients cannot tolerate the side effects of these drugs.

The newest addition to the glaucoma armamentarium is latanoprost (Xalatan). Instead of slowing the production of aqueous humor, it lowers intraocular pressure by increasing drainage of the fluid. It also increases the amount of brown pigmentation in the irises of about 7 percent of patients who use it, causing a gradual change in the color of their eyes.

The discovery that marihuana reduces intraocular pressure occurred accidentally during an experiment at UCLA designed to determine whether, as the Los Angeles Police Department believed, cannabis dilated the pupils. The police claimed that this supposed dilation (along with, among other things, white lips and a green-coated tongue) was a sign of marihuana intoxication and therefore good grounds for searching and arresting a citizen. The subjects of the experiment were normal volunteers smoking government-grown marihuana. Their eyes were photographed as they smoked, and the pupils were found to be slightly constricted rather than dilated. An ophthalmological examination showed that cannabis also reduced tearing (users have often claimed that they can comfortably chop onions while high) and intraocular pressure. Further experiments indicated a similar effect in patients with glaucoma. Marihuana reduced intraocular pressure for an average of four to five hours, with "no indications of any deleterious effects . . . on visual function or ocular structure."[9] Under its influence the pupils responded normally to light; visual acuity, refraction, peripheral visual fields, binocular vision, and color vision were not affected. The researchers concluded that marihuana may be more useful than conventional medications and probably works by a different mechanism. This conclusion has been confirmed by further human experiments and animal studies.

The effect on intraocular pressure occurs when marihuana is smoked or THC is taken orally. In one study nineteen patients smoked marihuana for thirty-five days and another twenty-nine patients smoked it for ninety-four days without developing tolerance to the effect on intraocular pressure or any deterioration of vision.[10] Several animal studies have established that cannabis is also active when applied topically (that is, as an eyedrop). This is important, because topical application has fewer psychological effects and is more acceptable to ophthalmologists. Unfortunately, cannabis preparations suitable for topical application in human beings have not yet been developed.

9. R. S. Hepler and I. M. Frank, "Marihuana Smoking and Intraocular Pressure," *JAMA* 217 (1971): 1392.

10. R. S. Hepler, I. M. Frank, and R. Petrus, "Ocular Effects of Marihuana Smoking," in *The Pharmacology of Marihuana*, ed. M. C. Braude and S. Szara, 2 vols. (New York: Raven, 1976), 2:815–824.

In the phase known as end-stage glaucoma, the patient has already lost a substantial degree of vision, the condition is worsening, standard drugs are no longer effective, and blindness is imminent. The writer of the following account, Robert Randall, had reached that stage when he began to smoke marihuana regularly as a medicine. He had used all the available glaucoma drugs at the highest permitted doses, and his intraocular pressure remained dangerously high. If nothing further had been done, he would have gone blind.

I smoked my first marihuana cigarette the day Richard Nixon was elected President. Jerry Ford was President when I smoked my first legal "research" joint. Jimmy Carter was elected days before I walked out of a Washington, D.C., hospital carrying the nation's first modern prescription for medical marihuana. I legally toked through the Reagan years, unscathed by the mindless War on Drugs. George Bush is President now. I still legally smoke medicinal marihuana and, as a result, still enjoy my sight.

My stepping stones to the wacky weed were alcohol and tobacco. I began smoking tobacco because I wanted to smoke pot and needed practice inhaling. A purely economic decision; tobacco then cost two cents a cigarette. Marihuana, by comparison, was obscenely expensive—fifteen to twenty dollars an ounce for the really good stuff. I was hooked on sweet nicotine after my first cigarette—an attraction I have yet to resolve.

Marihuana, of course, was profoundly different. It was far safer, nonaddictive, and illegal. Unlike many first time tokers I got blitzed. When I closed my eyes I saw glossy Kodachrome snaps—mental ViewMaster slides—of good friends looking very happy indeed. In another culture this might be interpreted as the weed's way of saying I needed the good it could afford. I enjoyed marihuana very much. It was fun.

My life underwent subtle, pervasive changes. First, an alteration in sensory inputs. Agonizingly loud, over-bright booze binges involving herds of highly intoxicated people were replaced by quiet evenings sitting in semi-darkness in a small circle of close confidants—fellow criminals against Empire all—listening to hard rock played low so as not to arouse suspicion, a towel stuffed under the door to avoid apprehension.

I cruised through college on clouds of cannabis, completed my undergraduate work early, and started my master's. No problems in the academy. Most of my friends smoked. I enjoyed smoking marihuana in groups or alone, learned to revel in the suddenly plastic character of thought. The marihuana-induced jump from hyper-linear sequencing to the universe of randomly interconnected thoughts and obtuse associations delighted me. McLuhan rendered comprehensible.

Finally, when I smoked marihuana I saw more clearly. I'm not talking enlightenment, I'm talking sight. Seeing. Since my mid-teens my evenings had been haunted by minor visual problems—transient tricolored halos. On some evenings I would go white-blind, my vision snared in an impenetrable swirl of absolute illumination—the white void.

I knew these problems were minor because when I mentioned them to my physicians they told me if I was older it might be serious. But, since I was too young for it to be serious it must be "eye strain." All that diligent study. If they weren't worried, why should I be? Particularly since marihuana relaxed my "eye strain." Nothing special in that. Marihuana relaxes nearly everything; mind, body, soul, that chronic kink in the neck. So why not eye strain? Without marihuana to ease my "eye strain" I probably could not have completed my master's.

Following graduation in 1971, I moved to Washington to write stirring speeches for powerful people and ended up driving a cab. I loved driving a cab. Most instructive. No boss. You set your own hours. I'd also stopped smoking marihuana. Being in a new city, surrounded by new people, I had few friends and no access—no dealer.

One evening in the summer of 1972, I closed my left eye and discovered I could not read with my right eye. Instead of clearly formed letters I saw a jumble of black ink splashed on a white page. No matter how close I drew the text, it remained indecipherable, incoherent, alien. Someone gave me the name of a good ophthalmologist. I saw him the following afternoon. I was twenty-four.

Benjamin Fine, M.D., one of the nation's leading ocular pathologists, performed a number of tests. I told him of my halos and white-blindness. His assistant took me through my first visual field examination. Eventually, the doctor called me to his inner office. There was grimness in his manner. Clearly, not good news.

Said Dr. Fine, "Son, you have a very serious condition called glaucoma. You have already suffered a lot of visual damage and . . ."

"How long?"

Thrown by my directness, he responded in kind: "At best you've got three, maybe five, years of remaining sight. You've lost most of the vision in both eyes. Your right eye has no central vision—no reading vision—none. In your left eye you only have a small island of healthy tissue. That's why you can read. Your pressure in both eyes is over forty. It should be under twenty. You are in very, very serious trouble. You are going to go blind."

Surgery was risky, especially in someone with my advanced level of damage. There was a good chance that surgery would annihilate the small fragments of healthy optic tissue that remained.

"I'm sorry, son. We'll do the best we can, but there's not a lot we can do. You are going to go blind." He looked worn out. Dr. Fine put pilocarpine in my eyes, gripped me by the shoulders, asked if I was all right, gave me a pat on the back, and sent me out the door with those most fateful words: "Just live life as you always have . . ." Patients know the end to this dreaded sentence, "because you won't have it for long."

Generally unfazed by this most pessimistic meeting on the future of my life, I wandered downstairs, got in my cab, and realized I could not see beyond the dashboard. Pilocarpine, a miotic, induces intense nearsightedness. I drove through D.C. rush-hour traffic guided by memory and the glare of sunlight off the cars in front of me.

I ignored this gaping invitation to debilitating depression. I could still see, still read, still softly fondle all nature's hues and tones. Until, of course, I put in my newly prescribed Pilo [pilocarpine], which quickly reduced my sight to remnants of ill-defined shape. My introduction to the wonderfully twisted world of glaucoma pharmacology.

Medically seeking to preserve sight by employing drugs that induce functional blindness results in what physicians disdainfully call "patient noncompliance." This means that if I really wanted to see a movie I'd stop taking Pilo, shrug off my pharmaceutically induced myopia, and enjoy the film.

Glaucoma and its therapies introduced me to much larger, more disruptive realities. Pilo and driving don't mix. Within a week of diagnosis I was out of my cab and out of work. Deemed "disabled," I landed on welfare, an unexpected ward of the state. This really was getting serious.

Within weeks of diagnosis my prescription for Pilo doubled, redoubled, tripled, quadrupled. Within months epinephrine was added. Epi caused my heart to race, opened my pupils wide, and let in such a flood of photons that I felt I was drowning in light. Then came Diamox [a carbonic anhydrase inhibitor], a pill, a diuretic. Crushing fatigue. The taste of everything changed. Finally, in desperation, phospholine iodide, an eyedrop developed from a World War II nerve gas, was added to the mix. This battering pharmaceutical assault left me blurry-eyed, dysfunctionally myopic, photophobic, extremely tired, with a chronic backache — from calcification of my kidneys. Objective medical control over elevated intraocular pressures (IOP), however, remained elusive. My rapidly escalating intake of toxic prescriptions was outraced by the dynamic character of my glaucoma. Each visual field shrank.

Despite my use of every pharmaceutical agent in the inventory, my evenings were routinely visited by tricolored halos — a signature of ocular pressures over 35 mm Hg [millimeters of mercury]. On some nights the halos were muted. On others they appeared as hard crystal rings emanating from every source of light.

And then there were nights, not so rare, of white-blindness—the world rendered invisible by its brilliance. Clinical translation: ocular tension in excess of 40 mm Hg. To summarize, things were not going very well.

Then someone gave me a couple of joints. Sweet weed! That night I made and ate dinner, watched television. My tricolored halos arrived, which made watching TV less interesting. So I put on some good music, dimmed offending lights, and got into some serious toking. I happened to look out my window at a distant street lamp and noticed what was not there. No halos. That's when I had the full-blown, omni-dimensional technicolor cartoon light-bulb experience. In a transcendent instant the spheres spoke! So simple. Old messages—new context. You smoke pot, your eye strain goes away. Ganja is good for you.

Sure was fun, but in the medicated haze of the next miotic morning I chided my raging rapture and began a baseline reality check. My well-educated, acutely dispassionate intellect was not kind. "Let us," my left sphere said, "be analytical." Brace yourself—the facts are not pretty. This poor, super-stressed soul, unwilling to accept the cumulative horror of what has become "real life," gets his hands on some really good pot. He smokes a couple of joints and gets a bit dopey. OK, certifiably Fruit Loops. In despair and desperation, he imagines marihuana is going to "save his sight."

Are we crazy? The answer is obvious, right? Given these facts, who would not want to believe that something mystical, magical, mysterious, and forbidden is going to rescue them from the pit of eternal darkness? The idea that a legally prohibited, medically unavailable weed—a plant smoked for sheer delight, for fun—is going to "save your sight" is madcap and reckless, as farfetched, improbable, and pathetic a notion as someone insane could imagine. So began six months of cynical observation. Six months of simple trial and error. At the end the conclusion was unavoidable. Without marihuana there were halos and white-blind nights. When I smoked marihuana there were no halos. Is a pattern emerging? You bet. If I watched very closely I could actually observe the halos depart. The cumulative evidence of a reproducible benefit was inescapable.

So, I accept that an illegal, medically prohibited weed may help me not to go blind. What now? Do I rush to introduce nice, middle-aged, middle-of-the-road, prestigious ocular pathologist and genuinely swell fellow Dr. Ben Fine to my pot-driven revelation, which is, of course, of potential benefit to millions of similarly afflicted humans? Yeah, right! No way! He's a good doctor. I like him. He's honest. But he would not appreciate my news. There are medical questions. And, of course, legal concerns. Like malpractice or worse. If Dr. Fine knows but does not tell the police, does he become my criminal accomplice? A co-conspirator? "Pot Doc arrested!" His career in ruins.

If not my trusted doctor, then whom? I could tell the drug bureaucrats? Sure! "Marihuana Can Be Good for You!" This is just the sort of good news rabid antidrug zealots are longing to hear. In this very unsubtle way, fear—prohibition-induced fear—pervades any dialogue on marihuana's medical use, separating patients from physicians, from other patients, from government. You are isolated. In the best of times, under the best of circumstances, this is not something to be wished for. When you are young and going blind, the inability to share such vital information with the physician treating you or with others who might be helped becomes downright scary. It became a time of simple goals. Keep smoking, keep your mouth shut, and stay sighted. Seeing is real. Everything else is politics.

Dr. Fine, though mystified by the sudden change in my condition, was greatly pleased by the results. My ever-eroding visual fields stabilized. My slide into darkness slowed, then halted. As my glaucoma came under medical management, other aspects of life began to right themselves. I escaped welfare and took a part-time teaching job at a local college.

Discounting unsavory encounters with underworld characters, illegal marihuana is frightfully expensive, absolutely unregulated, and not always available. To cope with the uncertainty of adequate supply I did what many patients still do. I grew some pot.

In 1974 I tried cultivating cannabis indoors, only to watch as devouring squadrons of spider mites euphorically consumed my entire crop. The next spring two small marihuana plants— the product of seeds unintentionally dropped the year before— sprouted through the boards of my sun deck. We re-potted the seeds, planted a few more, then watched nature do the rest. By midsummer we were blessed by beautiful six-foot pot plants. Things were going swell. My vision was stable. I was employed. I'd rediscovered loose change. Alice had come to live with me. Swell. These were the last quiet days of my life.

While we were vacationing in Indiana, the local vice cops raided my house and seized my six-foot marihuana plants. I returned to find a warrant on the kitchen table with a note scribbled on the back requesting that I surrender myself for arrest. I could not know this at the time, but being arrested was about the best thing that could have happened to me. Being arrested "saved my sight."

When I told my attorneys I was smoking marihuana to treat my glaucoma, they thought it was hysterical. When they realized I was not joking, they stopped laughing only long enough to tell me to "prove it." I spoke with Keith Stroup, head of the National Organization for the Reform of Marijuana Laws. Keith didn't laugh. Instead, he carefully explained that I didn't have a prayer. But he gave me a few phone numbers and suggested I call around. So I phoned around the federal bureaucracy. Needless to say, I was startled when at least three bureaucrats point-blank told me, "Oh, we know marihuana helps glaucoma. We have lots of data which shows . . ." They knew! They knew and hadn't bothered to tell me. They knew, but did not want anyone else to know. Remember, this is 1975, not yesterday.

Given a choice between administering a reckless, well-established, absolute, and catholic prohibition or honestly meeting the urgent medical needs of desperately ill citizens, the drug bureau-

crats had, of course, chosen deceit to maintain their institution-
ally treasured fraud. This is why bureaucrats the world 'round are
so beloved by the citizens they serve.

Proving that marihuana lowers intraocular pressures is not
difficult. The government, my government, was fully aware of
marihuana's beneficial effects on glaucoma by early 1971. Marihuana is a political issue, not a mere medical matter. Besides,
you cannot make a profit growing medicinal weeds. The medical
mandarins occupying the National Eye Institute did not wish to
get involved. They, too, were afraid. It might hurt funding. When
I requested help, NEI refused to conduct any experiments with
marihuana because I might want to use the data in court. The
nation's leading ocular specialists were politically correct and very
antimarihuana. Besides, the doctors said thoughtfully, you could
never use marihuana. Marihuana causes people to "get high."
And we all know just how life-threatening euphoria can be.

Eventually I underwent two highly controlled medical experiments. The first, conducted at the Jules Stein Eye Institute, UCLA,
required my incarceration in a mental ward for thirteen days of
round-the-clock observation. I arrived in the middle of an on-
going research project involving six "routine" research subjects
who were being tested on pure synthetic THC—a man-made
copy of marihuana's most mind-altering chemical. The UCLA researchers did more than simply confirm that marihuana lowered
my ocular tension. They discovered that my disease could not be
controlled using conventional glaucoma medicines. Left on these
drugs I would go blind, just as Dr. Fine predicted. I was also
tested on synthetic THC [Marinol]. What a lousy, marginal drug!
The "high" is anxiety-provoking. The therapeutic effects, if any,
are minimal, transient, unpredictable. But THC comes in a pill.
The bureaucrats, the research scientists and doctors can relate
to pills. Besides, we all know you shouldn't smoke. In the end
UCLA determined marihuana was not merely beneficial; it was
critical to the medical maintenance of my vision.

OK. It's proved. Let's go to court. I was ready, but my anxious attorneys conspired with an even more anxiety-ridden Dr. Fine to compel me into a second, confirmatory evaluation. On the Ides of March, 1976, a second, much less fun experiment was undertaken at the Wilmer Eye Institute at Johns Hopkins University, where I was institutionalized for six of the most miserable days of my existence. The Wilmer physicians were under strict instructions from Dr. Fine to find a conventional solution. He didn't want to testify in court. So they threw every glaucoma drug in the book at my condition. I wandered into the medical library, where I became alarmed by the cumulative adverse effects commonplace among chronic users of glaucoma medicines. A brief list would include cataracts, kidney stones, gastric ulcers, skin rashes, drug fevers, mental confusion, abrupt mood swings, hypertension, renal, respiratory, or cardiac failure, death. The Wilmer Eye Institute physicians, despite their seemingly perverse glee in exposing me to highly toxic medicines, could not conduct an evaluation of marihuana. No government clearance. No grant.

In the midst of this meanness a most curious thing happened. I got to know my roomie, a fifty-three-year-old West Virginia factory worker named Vince. We had just met, barely exchanged hellos, when Vince asked, "You tried any good marihuana?" Blown away?! You bet. Seems ole Vince had taken a break with a couple of his night shift buddies and smoked weed for the first time in his life. Bingo! Vince noticed that his halos went away. "If I could get my hands on enough marihuana, I sure as hell wouldn't be in here," Vince convincingly said. Two days later I watched the guys in white wheel Vince into cryosurgery, a ghastly, painful procedure which freezes, kills, a part of the eye in an effort to reduce ocular pressure. That night Vince groaned in agony, his toes curled in torment. After leaving Wilmer I followed Vince's progress for quite some time. The mutilating surgery had not helped him. Eventually, unable to "get enough marihuana," Vince went blind.

I had been in glaucoma therapy for nearly four years, and Vince was the first glaucoma patient I'd ever met. And Vince knew!

How many others knew? At the conclusion of their pharmaceutical torment the Wilmer doctors grudgingly conceded failure. UCLA's evaluation was correct: in the absence of marihuana my ocular tension was beyond medical control. Ignoring the UCLA data on marihuana, the Wilmer surgeons recommended immediate surgical intervention.

What a surprise! Without marihuana I would go blind. Everyone agreed on that. The Wilmer physicians, in their zeal to evade this fact, had recommended surgical procedures Dr. Fine knew would result in blindness. He finally agreed to testify in my defense. He took the very highest ground; given the facts, it would be medically unethical to withhold marihuana. The rest, as they say, is history. Briefly summarized:

- In May 1976, I petitioned federal drug agencies for immediate access to government supplies of marihuana.
- In July, at my trial, we raised the untried legal defense of "medical necessity." Essentially, a simple argument that any sane soul who is going blind would break the law to save his sight.
- In November 1976, the bureaucrats cracked. They delivered a tin of three hundred pre-rolled marihuana cigarettes to my new doctor, John Merritt, at Howard University. In this way I became the first American to gain legal, medically supervised access to marihuana.
- In the same month, the D.C. Superior Court ruled that my use of marihuana was not criminal but an act of "medical necessity." It was the first successful articulation of the "medical necessity" defense in the history of English common law.

My first year of legal smoking was not tranquil. In fact it turned into a running battle. I'd speak out, the bureaucrats would try to clamp down. Very unpleasant. Increasing news coverage unhinged the bureaucrats. Other patients were expecting help. By early 1978, the feds hit the wall, bit the bullet, and cut off my legal line of supply. I countered by suing. Twenty-four hours after the suit was filed we arrived at an out-of-court settlement which is still in effect. This settlement assures me of medically appropriate (nonresearch) access to marihuana to meet my legitimate therapeutic needs.

Robert Randall was told by his ophthalmologists that he would be blind by the mid-1970s. He has been smoking marihuana since the early 1970s (from 1976 to the present legally with a Compassionate IND). He still (1996) has his eyesight.

Elvy Musikka is a woman in her mid-forties who lives in Hollywood, Florida. This is her story:

> In late February 1975 I went to see Dr. Rosenthal, a general practitioner in the Ft. Lauderdale area. He concluded a very thorough examination and said my eyes had been stricken with glaucoma. My [intraocular fluid] pressures were in the high 40s [pressure in the low teens is normal], and Dr. Rosenthal insisted I see an ophthalmologist immediately. His suspicions were confirmed, and I was started on pilocarpine eyedrops.
>
> By the spring of 1976 the pilocarpine itself was becoming a problem. I began seeing circles but assumed they were a symptom of the glaucoma. Wearing contact lenses was uncomfortable, and my pressures were going up. A new doctor suggested I consider marihuana because it was likely that otherwise I would go blind. He told me this as a friend, not a doctor; it was then that I began to realize that sometimes doctors have to choose between the Hippocratic oath and hypocritical laws. I was most fortunate that this man had a heart.
>
> Blindness was not new to me. I was born blind, with congenital cataracts, and had my first eye surgery at five. Surgery then was very different from the laser surgery of today, and I was left with a lot of scar tissue. I wore very thick glasses until fourteen or so, when I had surgery on my left eye. Something went wrong, and I lost most of my sight in that eye. But with 20/200 vision in the right eye and the help of contact lenses I had gotten along quite well, until this most recent finding.
>
> I was uncomfortable with the thought of taking marihuana, a

drug I had been misinformed to believe was as dangerous and addictive as heroin. Because of my anxiety, the first time I used it I became sick to my stomach. I find that particularly amusing now, as I have discovered that it is very effective in preventing and alleviating nausea. I have also discovered that, like myself at first, some people feel paranoid after using marihuana, but now I wonder whether this is an effect of the plant itself or due to longstanding myths about its dangerousness. I don't get paranoid using it any more—maybe that is a clue?

That summer I discovered something curious. One day I visited the doctor, scared to death because my friend Jerry and I had spent an awful lot of the night before drinking champagne. I presumed it would have increased my pressures and was very surprised to find that they were twelve and thirteen. My doctor explained that downers such as alcohol, marihuana, and Demerol bring pressures down. He felt the safest of the three was marihuana.

I was having a terrible time smoking it, so my doctor and I decided it would be best for me to take it in brownies instead. He warned I would need a bit more than smoking. He gave me a recipe that called for an ounce of marihuana to yield a batch of twenty-four brownies—a twelve-day supply.

I didn't know where to go for marihuana and didn't always have access to it. Once my pressures were so high my doctor obtained some for me. It was handled through his secretary. Oh, that poor woman! How she shook! Her hands were ice cold when she handed me the bag. I thanked God for these compassionate people. I knew the street value was thirty to forty dollars an ounce but she took only fifteen dollars. That couldn't continue, of course, and I sought to obtain marihuana legally.

I couldn't find enough and had to keep using pilocarpine. When it started making me see circles again, my doctor was out of town, and I went to a new clinic. When the attending physician there realized that I was using marihuana to treat my glaucoma, he looked very disgusted. He threw two prescriptions at me and sent me home without instructions and warnings. Those two drugs were the most horrible I have ever come across in my life. Diamox took all the potassium out of my body and left me completely apathetic. My children had to care for themselves because when I came home I could only go to bed. At the time I did not have the money to buy the second prescription, phospholine iodide, which I eventually tried and found unbearably painful.

I called my hometown newspaper and told a reporter about my use of marihuana in a telephone interview. I spoke without giving my name or picture, because I feared losing my job and custody of my children. But a lot of people recognized the story as mine and came forward, confessing that they were regular marihuana smokers and would help me get marihuana when possible. You can imagine my shock! Some of these people were co-workers, others respected members of the community. None of them—not a one—was a bum, as I had been led to think of every marihuana smoker.

In January 1977 my doctor sent me to a research center at the University of Miami. He thought they might help me obtain marihuana legally. But the very dedicated scientists at the center didn't want to hear the "m" word. Instead I spent one of the most grueling days of my life. When I arrived my pressures were in the high 50s in the right eye and the high 40s in the left. They gave me everything they could think of. Drops didn't help much, nor did using a little pump to flush the eye. I also had to drink a big glass of a sickeningly sweet liquid, which didn't help either. At the day's end my pressures had barely lowered to the 40s, so I was scheduled for emergency surgery.

At home that night I used a remaining bit of marihuana to bake some brownies and ate one every twelve hours. The doctors were shocked when they checked my pressures as I arrived for surgery the next Monday morning—perfectly normal at 14 and 16! Regardless, they readied me for surgery, even though it had at best a 30 percent chance of helping me! The following morning they performed an operation on my tear ducts which turned out to be of no value. Because of it I now have to wear the big magnifying glasses that I had managed to avoid since childhood. After this procedure I had less sight, more scar tissue, and higher pressures, and I was unable to return to work.

I now faced not only glaucoma but depression and poverty. It would be at least nine months before Social Security could issue a disability check. I was humiliated in using food stamps but glad they were available. I developed insomnia. Marihuana was harder to find now that I had no money to buy it. Sometimes compassionate people gave me some and my insomnia disappeared. It was certainly the best antidepressant I have ever come across.

By 1980 I had little money, and marihuana had gone up in price, so I started growing my own plants. I used the finest seeds, which produced small plants, hard to detect but productive. I required only three or four joints a day. My pressures became so close to normal that my doctors decided a corneal transplant was safe. It worked! I never have had such beautiful eyesight—it was so wonderful! I was so happy, until neighbors jumped the fence around my yard and stole my marihuana plants.

My pressures went sky high, and I escaped into alcohol quite a bit of the time. When I started having slight blackouts I realized that alcohol was not the answer. So reluctantly and fearfully I went through surgery again. This time I hemorrhaged, and before I knew it, my right eye was blind. Since I had only 20/400 vision in my left eye, you could have lit up my bedroom with bright lights as I slept and I wouldn't have awakened. I was very depressed. Most painful were the happy dreams in which I was seeing out of both eyes and being the person I used to be. Then I would wake up to find myself without the right eye.

I needed money and had an extra room in my house, so I put an ad in the paper and acquired a boarder. He assured me he was not taking illegal drugs and would not tell anyone I was growing marihuana. But soon his erratic behavior convinced me there was a problem, and sure enough, I found cocaine under the bathroom sink. At first he denied using drugs, but a few days later he admitted it. He said he needed cocaine because in his job as a car salesman he was expected to work seven days a week, ten hours a day. I told him that I didn't care about his reasons; he would have to move. He agreed that he would, but as the time grew closer he became reluctant. We argued, and he turned me in to the police.

I was arrested on the night of March 4, 1988, and it changed my life forever. I notified the media, and this time my hometown paper photographed me and wrote a full follow-up story. I was contacted by people who had obtained marihuana legally, and my doctor and his secretary spent at least fifty hours on paperwork to be submitted to the DEA, FDA, and NIDA in an effort to secure legal marihuana. I did a lot of radio shows, and it was always heartbreaking because almost always there was someone who had lost their sight unnecessarily. There were also genuinely concerned citizens who worried about my being addicted to a horrible drug and who sincerely wished that there was another answer for me. Of course, they weren't me and hadn't been on it for twelve years, so they didn't realize that there were no side effects for me to fear. I began to hear from people all over the country, even some from Canada. It was amazing; many were glaucoma patients who had maintained their sight for twenty and twenty-five years with marihuana and are still illegally maintaining it today. I envied them for standing up for their health, for knowing what they were doing and taking care of themselves.

But that was no help to me now. I was facing felony charges. In Florida, possession of anything over twenty grams is a felony, and they confiscated an ounce and a half from a plant I had just harvested the previous Monday.

My trial began and ended August 15, 1988. I knew one thing: if I was going to court, so was this unjust law. I was not afraid. I felt that God and his angels were with me. I was not mistaken — the only person they could find to testify against me was the arresting officer, and I wouldn't say he was against me. Glaucoma patients testified on my behalf, and my doctor proclaimed marihuana the only agent that ever provided reliable relief for me. I was asked if I had smoked marihuana since my arrest and I answered yes. "Did you smoke marihuana today?" "Of course," I replied. The judge listened carefully and decided that for me not to have tried to preserve whatever sight I had left would have been total insanity. He said that I had no intent of criminal activity, and I was acquitted. I had applied for a Compassionate IND in March 1988 and was granted legal use of marihuana provided by the government beginning October 21, 1988.

The sight in my right eye is coming back. I now have perceptions of light, colors, and shapes. In my left eye, which used to be 20/400 but is now 20/100, the optic nerve is very healthy and I have lost no peripheral vision. As a matter of fact it has improved. Miraculous—that's cannabis.

Some patients discontinue conventional glaucoma medicines altogether in favor of cannabis. Harvey J. Ginsburg, Ph.D., who wrote the following account, added marihuana to the regimen prescribed by his ophthalmologist:

I am a forty-seven-year-old professor of psychology at Southwest Texas State University and a current project director for the National Science Foundation. My wife, Diana, was, until recently, the special education counselor at San Marcos High School in San Marcos, Texas. On June 24, 1994, we were both arrested for felony possession of marihuana—six plants and eight ounces of marihuana brownies. A teenager who was an acquaintance of my son had placed an anonymous call to the local police for a $1,000 reward, responding to a Crimestoppers advertisement that offered "a profitable, exciting, guilt-free way to earn money."

Since 1980 I have been suffering from open-angle glaucoma, a disorder that runs in my family. Between 1980 and 1994 I took a number of prescription medications, including Timoptic, Betoptic [timolol and betaxolol, beta-blockers], Ocusert [pilocarpine], and Propine [dipivefrine, another topical glaucoma drug]. In 1986, after reading the scientific literature, I also began to grow and use marihuana.

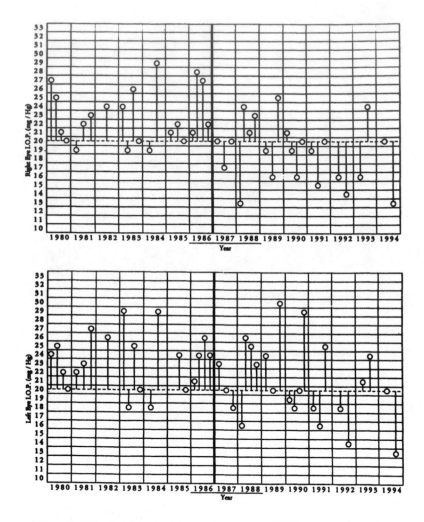

Figure 1. Right and left eye intra-ocular pressure (IOP) measurements (mm Hg) 1980–1986 (prescription medications only) and 1987–1994 (prescription medications plus marihuana).

The chart shows my intraocular pressure (IOP). Measures were taken regularly by an ophthalmologist, usually four times a year, from 1980 to 1994. Figure 1 shows the difference marihuana made. Before I started to use it only 17 percent of readings in the right eye and 10 percent in the left eye gave a pressure below 20 mg of mercury. After I started using it the pressure fell to below 20 mg in 52 percent of the right eye readings and 39 percent of the left eye readings.

Maybe the condition would have improved without marihuana, but that seems doubtful given the nature of glaucoma. Certainly the prescription medications I was taking were not preventing progression of the disease, as my ophthalmologist has testified. The addition of new prescription drugs might have achieved the same result, but until the federal research prohibition on marihuana is lifted, this plausible rival hypothesis cannot be tested. I can only say now that 2 grams of marihuana per day, in combination with other drugs, showed long-term effectiveness in reducing the high intraocular pressure associated with my open-angle glaucoma.

While I prepared to present a defense of medical necessity at my trial, the district attorney had the state comptroller file a lien against our property and freeze our assets to enforce payment of the Texas Controlled Substances tax, $2,450 penalty and interest. The U.S. Supreme Court has ruled a similar tax in Montana unconstitutional. After learning of my medical condition, the comptroller's agent who took the tax money from me shook her head and asked, "When are these laws going to change?"

On July 31, 1995, the DA moved to dismiss all charges against us, and the judge agreed. A week later the San Marcos chief of police wrote an angry letter to the town's newspaper expressing his displeasure. Then the local police decided to impose their own vigilante "justice." The chief's captain of narcotics contacted the school superintendent, who threatened to fire Diana and try to get her teaching license revoked on the grounds that she had violated the district's zero-tolerance policy by living with an accused marihuana user. Diana eventually did resign, although she got a favorable out-of-court settlement from the school district.

In the absence of marihuana, my IOP initially showed an unexpected dramatic decrease but then increased to the highest level ever. As a result, my ophthalmologist prescribed yet another drug, Ocupress [carteolol—a beta-blocker]. The FDA has approved it despite potential side effects that include stroke and cardiac arrest. Another recently approved medication, Xalatan [latanoprost], turns blue eyes permanently brown by a mechanism that is completely unknown and may eventually create health problems as well. Marihuana's safety and its capacity to reduce intraocular pressure are well known, yet federal and state governments persist in their zero-tolerance policy, while law enforcement agents and other government officials wonder why ordinary citizens are becoming increasingly hostile to them. The tax agent's question remains: When are these laws going to change?

EPILEPSY

Epilepsy is a condition in which certain brain cells (the epileptic focus) become abnormally excitable and spontaneously discharge in an uncontrolled way, causing a seizure. In grand mal or generalized epilepsy, the abnormal cells are on both sides of the brain and the discharge produces convulsions (violent muscle spasms). In absence seizures, the generalized brain discharge causes a lapse of consciousness but not convulsions. Partial seizures result from abnormal discharge in an isolated area of the brain and may occur with or without a change in consciousness.

Partial seizures with a change in consciousness, known as complex partial seizures, are caused by damage to the temporal or frontal lobes of the cerebral cortex. They were formerly known as psychomotor seizures because the symptoms also include motor activity (grimacing and repetitive mouth or hand movements are especially common). When overexcitation is confined to a very small area, the patient with epilepsy may have a strange sensation of déjà vu, vertigo, fear, or an odd smell without a source. This experience, known as an aura, may or may not be followed by a full, complex, partial seizure.

Epilepsy is treated mainly with anticonvulsant drugs, including carbamazepine (Tegretol), phenytoin (Dilantin), valproic acid (Depakote), phenobarbital, primidone (Mysoline), ethosuximide (Zarontin), and clonazepam (Klonopin). About 70 percent of patients get relief from one of these drugs, and another 10 percent are helped by some combination of them.[11] Focal seizures and temporal lobe epilepsy, however, often respond poorly to these drugs.[12] Furthermore, anticonvulsants have many potentially serious side effects, including bone softening, anemia, swelling of the gums, double vision, hair loss, headaches, nausea, decreased libido, impotence, depression, and psychosis. Overdoses or idiosyncratic reactions may lead to loss of motor coordination, coma, and even death.[13]

Although the anticonvulsant properties of cannabis have been known since ancient times and were explored in the nineteenth century, this therapeutic use of the drug has been largely ignored in the past hundred years. A rare exception is a short paper by J. P. Davis and H. H. Ramsey published in 1949. They studied the effects of two tetrahydrocannabinol congeners on five institutionalized children with severe grand mal epilepsy that was inadequately controlled by the standard anticonvulsant drugs, phenobarbital and phenytoin (Dilantin). Three did no worse than before; the fourth became almost completely free of seizures and the fifth entirely so.[14]

The medical literature was again silent on this topic until 1975, when the following case of grand mal epilepsy was reported:

A twenty-four-year-old man has been seen in a neurology outpatient clinic for a period of eight years for control of his epileptic

11. M. J. Brodie and M. A. Dichter, "Antiepileptic Drugs," *New England Journal of Medicine*, Review Article 334:3 (Jan. 18, 1996): 168–175.

12. P. Robb, "Focal Epilepsy: The Problem, Prevalence, and Contributing Factors," *Advanced Neurology* 8 (1975): 11–22.

13. H. Kutt and S. Louis, "Untoward Effects of Anticonvulsants," *New England Journal of Medicine* 286 (1972): 1316–1317.

14. J. P. Davis and H. H. Ramsey, "Antiepileptic Action of Marijuana-active Substances," *Federation Proceedings* 8 (1949): 284–285.

seizures. His history included febrile convulsions at three years of age and epileptic seizures since the age of sixteen. Since that age the patient has been taking diphenylhydantoin sodium (phenytoin), 100 mg four times a day, and phenobarbital, 30 mg four times a day. Control of seizures with this regimen was incomplete, and the patient complained of attacks about once every two months. From the age of sixteen to twenty-two, the incidence of seizures increased from one attack per month to one per week.

At twenty-two years of age the patient began smoking marihuana (two to five joints per night) while continuing the prescribed anticonvulsant drug therapy. During this period, attacks did not occur as long as the patient continued to take the combination of all three drugs. The patient's condition could not be maintained on marihuana alone, because on two occasions he experienced an attack three to four days after running out of his prescribed medication.[15]

In a later study, sixteen patients with grand mal epilepsy who were not responding well to treatment were given 200 to 300 milligrams of cannabidiol or a placebo in addition to their antiepileptic drugs. After five months, three of the cannabidiol patients showed complete improvement, two exhibited partial improvement, and two showed minor improvement; one was unchanged. Mild sedation was the only side effect. Of the placebo patients, only one improved substantially, and seven were unchanged. The researchers concluded that for some patients, cannabidiol combined with standard antiepileptics may be useful in controlling seizures. Whether cannabidiol alone in large doses would be helpful is not known.[16]

Although the medical establishment is still showing little interest, more and more epilepsy sufferers are discovering the usefulness of cannabis. Carl Oglesby has a complex partial seizure disorder; the

15. P. F. Consroe, G. C. Wood, and H. Buchsbaum, "Anticonvulsant Nature of Marihuana Smoking," *JAMA* 234 (1975): 306–307.

16. J. M. Cunha, E. A. Carlini, A. E. Pereira, et al., "Chronic Administration of Cannabidiol to Healthy Volunteers and Epileptic Patients," *Pharmacology* 21 (1980): 175–185.

seizure arises in the temporal lobe and spreads, but remains relatively focal.

In 1972, at the age of thirty-seven, I discovered that marihuana medicated a seizure that had plagued me since my teenage years and for which no legal medication seemed available. Shortly after that I became a daily user. Today, because I am uncomfortable with the legal risks of using marihuana, I am resolved to find a different way to deal with my problem.

My seizure first appeared when I was fifteen or sixteen and has persisted to my current age of fifty-four at a rate varying from a half dozen to two dozen episodes a day. Episodes vary in duration (from a half minute to a minute) and in intensity, but never in form. There are always two stages. The first is an onset or aura stage, and the second is defined by the facial spasm that forms the crux of the seizure.

The first warning comes as a subtle yet ineffably corporeal sensation, an uh-oh feeling, distinctly unpleasant, of lightness and airiness, a kind of inner tickling with a throbbing, giddy quality. It is centered in my chest at first, but diffuses into my head within a few seconds and incorporates the entire background of mental activity. That is, I can still talk and sustain a line of thought, but it requires special effort because of an inclusive if private sense of alarm.

I am aware of some physical displays that I cannot control during the onset. My nostrils flare, my eyes dance and sparkle, my voice tightens and its pitch becomes erratic, my diaphragm contracts, my breathing becomes irregular, and I feel vaguely disoriented. It is as though my body becomes excited, almost pleasantly so, but without any social or mental correlative, context, or motive. Since the loss of physical control over oneself is always disconcerting, an experience that bears a certain gross resemblance to glee becomes a source of helplessness and dread.

The seizure proper emerges as a crescendo from the aura and is partly an intensification of the aura. Its dominant component, however, is a physically irresistible grin that takes over the entire right side of my face without affecting the left side at all. Everything else about the seizure, as far as I can tell, is bilateral: both eyes sparkle, both sides of my diaphragm contract, both nostrils flare. But this uniformly right-sided rictus is the ground zero of the seizure, the point and climax toward which the aura phase ascends. The aura stage is essentially private and easily concealed, but the rictus subjects me to social penalties. I can conceal it only by hiding my face or diverting attention from myself.

When the seizure first appeared I could not understand or explain it and felt too ashamed to ask for help. My parents, unsophisticated people, reprimanded me for what my father called my "silly grin" (as in "get that silly grin off your face"). When I tried to explain it to my friends, they responded that I should laugh if I felt like laughing. I couldn't make them understand that I didn't feel like laughing—or that, perhaps, yes, I did, but the feeling came over me as though from elsewhere and had no connection with any thought or perception or ordinary motivation. I could not convey this sense of externality, of being seized by a motive beyond consciousness.

So I gave up, resolved to keep this shameful thing, my silly grin, as much to myself as possible, and developed a repertoire of concealments. I credit myself with not becoming reclusive. I debated in high school and college, took up work that kept me in constant contact with other people, and later, in my early thirties, played a leading role (as president of Students for a Democratic Society, SDS) in opposing the Vietnam War. I even performed on stage for several years in college and loved it, although I eventually had to concede that the seizure made acting impossible.

If a seizure threatened at an inopportune moment—which happened constantly—I had a variety of responses. If I was holding the floor, I would divert attention from myself somehow, often simply by asking someone a question. If necessary I would stage a little choking fit, pick up a glass of water, and use it as a prop to help conceal the rictus. In other settings I might conveniently discover a piece of apple stuck in an upper molar on the right side of my mouth. I let only my most intimate friends know that I had a problem.

As I grew older and provisionally more sophisticated, I came across theories that seemed to offer an explanation or at least an interpretation of my seizure, notably the popularized Freudianism that was so inescapable in the fifties and sixties. For a long time I adopted the view that my silly grin was psychosomatic in origin and I could get to the bottom of it, and perhaps cure it, only through psychoanalysis. Before I could explore this possibility, however, I was persuaded by a medical doctor in whom I confided (a) that the seizure was probably a kind of epilepsy and (b) that my means of coping with it were probably as sound as anything formal medicine could supply.

Like many others in the 1960s, I repeatedly came into contact with marihuana, but for several years I resisted the temptation to smoke it. I was highly visible as an SDS national officer and felt obliged to avoid bringing the organization into disrepute; besides, SDS had taken a strong anti marihuana position at my urging. Finally, unlike most rank-and-file members of the movement, I was a family man and the father of three children toward whom I felt a parent's normal responsibilities as those were understood in the American 1950s.

But in 1970 or thereabouts, with SDS destroyed, leadership of the antiwar movement in other hands, and my paternal pretensions the victims of divorce and separation, my curiosity won out and I began to experiment with marihuana in social situations. I soon discovered that my seizures vanished when I was high. After a few puffs, the aura and its ascent to the dreaded rictus simply did not occur for two to three hours.

I also enjoyed pleasures of the marihuana high itself. In sharp contradistinction to alcohol, it was no threat to self-control, and in fact improved my ability to speak extemporaneously. That alone would never have led me to become a regular user, since I was always unhappy about the idea of smoking. But marihuana's power to eliminate my seizures led me to adopt it as a regular medication. Several months ago I resolved to abandon this form of self-medication and simply suffer the consequences—more tolerable to me now than in 1970 because I am much less often called upon to speak in public (I still give perhaps a dozen public lectures a year). Nevertheless, the return of the seizures is saddening and to a certain extent dispiriting, so I have sought professional medical help in the hope of finding a workable, safe, and legal alternative.

Gordon Hanson is a fifty-three-year-old man who suffers from both grand mal epilepsy and absence attacks. These were partially controlled with the standard drugs phenytoin (Dilantin), primidone (Mysoline), and phenobarbital, but there were serious side effects. Here is his account:

Thinking back to the years before high school graduation is much easier for me than thinking about what happened after that chilly day in September 1956. Northerly winds scattered the fallen leaves as I hurried to fill my bucket with bright red cranberries against the setting sun of a shorter day. My emotions were mixed; this was my first season free of school, but I was uncertain of the future. On that September evening I felt very sleepy and retired before 10 P.M. Awakening was a revolving point of confusion and depression followed by nausea, headache, and muscle soreness that seemed to cover my entire body. My family surrounded the bed, their faces filled with concern. As soon as daylight came I was hurried to see our family doctor in Baudette. His diagnosis made me feel even more frightened and frustrated. How could I have epilepsy?

The affliction was kept as much a secret as possible. As the years passed, unpredictable petit mal seizures made an appearance, while the less frequent grand mal continued its haunting signs of approach—sounds of no meaning or apparent source, inability to speak, and finally the creeping paralysis that slowly engulfed my body. Unconsciousness would hide any injury until

I once again regained my senses. Burns and broken bones were not uncommon, yet not as foreboding as the lingering deep depression.

Combinations of prescription drugs, including Dilantin, Mysoline, and phenobarbital, did decrease the number of seizures but definitely did not cure the problems. Deep sadness would often overwhelm my life for days. Epilepsy was naturally assumed to be the cause—no one ever told me then that the drugs used to prevent seizures also had bad side effects. I drank alcohol for a few years, but it proved to be such a short-lived escape. Finally I met a girl I wanted to marry, but because I was afraid she would reject me, I did not tell her of my epileptic problems before our marriage.

Our youth and her gift of a daughter shielded us from pain for a short time. But the necessities of survival became ever more difficult to obtain, and the seizures became more frequent. My wife began to use alcohol to hide herself from a person she had now begun to fear because of the strange seizures and lingering mood swings that created a Jekyll-Hyde syndrome. Her drinking and my response to it increased our unhappiness, which was relieved only for a short time by the birth of another daughter and a son in the early sixties. My seizures and financial problems increased.

At the end of the sixties I had many confrontations with the law. In the early seventies the children were temporarily removed from our home. The court told me to consult a marriage counselor, who suggested I might try marihuana to decrease the depressive effect of phenobarbital and still control the seizures. This seemed absurd to me, as my attitude was the same as the majority's: this was a drug only whispered about, definitely evil!

Thank God, I began to read about the plant and also made inquiries to other sources, including the University of Minnesota. I found out that it had been used medically in centuries gone by, and I began to smoke it regularly.

By 1976 I cut my dose of phenobarbital, Dilantin, and Mysoline by about 50 percent. Seizures had become less frequent and mood swings had dwindled, at least when marihuana was available. In 1976 I was arrested for possession of a small amount, and after that I found it harder to purchase. The judge asked me to consult a doctor. The doctor didn't deny the medical usefulness of marihuana, but because it was illegal, he suggested I take Valium. For nearly two years I took two Valium pills a day, but it made a walking zombie of me, and I still had blackouts.

In 1978 my wife was hospitalized for three days after she mistook phenobarbital for aspirin while intoxicated. That made me discard my remaining phenobarbital and Valium completely. My mind was clear after withdrawal. I decided to try growing plants from accumulated seed that spring. It was rather successful. With each new year came new methods for better quality, leaving unpleasant memories behind. By 1982 I was growing enough in my garden to reduce my use of prescription drugs even further. Grand mal seizures had vanished, and the petit mal seizures numbered less than ten a year. Unfortunately, that summer I found the law frowning on my harvest of the herb, and I was arrested for possession of what they called a large amount. I continued to grow plants while awaiting the outcome of a long court battle that ended in 1985 with a two-month jail sentence. I was given more pills, but I still had seizures in jail. Another drug, Tranxene [clorazepate, an antianxiety drug and muscle relaxant related to Valium] was prescribed, but I used very little because I realized that the effects were similar to Valium.

On release I again started to use marihuana for relief from the pills and the blackouts. Our family life became pleasant as the years slipped gently by. An average growth of forty hemp plants supplied by nature decreased my need for man-made chemicals to one dose of Dilantin and one dose of Mysoline a day. Petit mal seizures now occurred five times a year or less, mostly in winter when I ran out of marihuana. Life became much more harmonious.

In 1988 there was a drought, my marihuana was stunted, and I was forced to buy off the street only four months after harvest.

The street price had risen so high I could barely afford it. Friends helped me until the next growing season, but I still had many seizures when marihuana was unavailable. Determined not to be caught short again, in 1989 I planted three times as many marihuana plants, each trimmed to resemble a short bushy tomato plant.

In late July I pulled up a couple and put them in our old vacant barn to dry. The rest of the story is a disaster—five police officers kicking in my front door before 6 A.M. and holding my wife, my son, and myself at gunpoint. My son lost his job because he wasn't allowed to leave for work that morning. Needless to say, all the marihuana was taken. After paying a bond, I was released, only to relive the experience in my dreams each night for weeks. My life since that day has been an experiment that resolves my doubts about the medical value of marihuana. Because of its unavailability I have suffered nearly two hundred seizures, including several of the grand mal type.

On June 22, 1991, what I had feared happened. A telephone call from my attorney in Minneapolis informed me that I had to report to Roseau County Jail for a sentence of six months. The Minnesota Supreme Court had denied my appeal. Now I sit in a cell with no provisions for personal safety. The cell is isolated. I have no way to communicate with the jailer's office, and the two prisoners I share it with have not been told what to do if a seizure should occur.

It is strange to think back to the early 1970s when I was told to consult a marriage counselor who advised me to use marihuana instead of prescription drugs. Now the law has taken me away from my wife and put me in prison because I complied with that suggestion, which had been successful in controlling my seizures and bringing love back to us. Now the law is once more forcing prescription drugs on me. I fear the dreaded cumulative side effects will return and cause me to become that nightmarish creature who brought so much grief to my wife and family. I cannot expect her to accept such a situation again after the solution we

achieved by discovering God's creation of such a wondrous healing herb. Apparently my only alternative is to use no drugs at
all when I am released. This will cause much unnecessary hard-
ship not only for me but also for my wife, who will have to
contend with the seizures and the depressive moods that follow.
I can only pray that our government will recognize marihuana's
medical uses before my release. If not, I cannot expect Connie to
accept me home.

Valerie Corral is a forty-four-year-old horticulturist who has organized a medical marihuana cooperative, the Wo·Men's Alliance for
Medical Marihuana (WAMM). Her interest in the issue comes from
personal experience:

The first day of spring in 1973 in the desert surrounding Pyra-
mid Lake, Nevada, was like any other March afternoon. Heat
rose from the earth in a snakelike dance as my friend and I drove
southwest from the lake after a long soak in the hot springs. It is
an exquisite land, an unearthly place, a reservation belonging to
the Paiute Indians.

As we cruised along Highway 445 an airplane swooped down
close to our Volkswagen. It was a P51 Mustang, a converted
World War II fighter. The plane came so near that we could see
the pilot's moustache. On its second pass it created a vortex that
caused us to lose control, skid, and roll for over 350 feet. My
friend and I were thrown out of the car and badly injured. She
was hospitalized with innumerable fractures, and I was left with
head injuries that caused grand mal seizures, sometimes as many
as five a day.

Becoming an epileptic changed my dreams and my destiny.
I would never again function as I had before. Frightened and
overwhelmed by the illness, I became a stranger to myself. I
was taking an array of antiepilepsy drugs that included Mysoline
[primidone], Dilantin [phenytoin], and phenobarbital. For pain
I was taking Percodan [a combination of oxycodone, an opioid,
and aspirin] and Valium [diazepam, an antianxiety drug]. I became an emotional cripple, physically dependent and under the

influence twenty-four hours a day, three hundred and sixty-five days a year. I stumbled through an ever-present drug haze in a futile attempt to control the spasms. I took more and more drugs, but only had more and more seizures.

The pharmaceutical delirium continued for two years. Although I was never diagnosed as psychotic, my behavior could be described that way. My body was also devastated. My gums began to swell and my white blood cell count plummeted. I had no resistance to infections; if I caught a cold, I risked a hospital stay. I could not be left alone; once I almost drowned after having a seizure in the bathtub. I did not want to live this wretched life in a drugged state. I knew that the FDA might never help me become seizure-free. I had to reconstruct my life to deal with my illness.

My husband, Mike, read in a medical periodical that laboratory-induced seizures in rats had been successfully controlled with marihuana. I had exhausted the pharmacopoeia of standard anti-epileptic drugs and was willing to try anything that might offer hope. I wanted what I thought to be a miracle. I wanted a normal life. In the spring of 1975 Mike and I moved to an isolated Santa Cruz mountaintop and opted to try marihuana in place of the antiepilepsy medicines. We planted seeds from several varieties that we had purchased and began experimenting.

After trying out "cold turkey" drug withdrawal—a method I do not recommend—I decided, with Mike's help, to withdraw gradually. For the next two and a half years, as I cut my medication with premeditated caution, I never traveled anywhere without a rolled joint. I smoked every day and took a puff whenever I felt an aura. I told my physician what I was doing, and he gave his tacit approval. Eventually I found that I could control the seizures completely with marihuana alone. We grew my medicine openly in our garden with our vegetables, herbs, and fruits. I seldom have to visit the physician any longer. I still have some neurological problems, but marihuana continues to alleviate the worst effects of my epilepsy without the side effects of the drugs I used to take.

In the late 1970s marihuana growing became a lucrative private enterprise, and the authorities escalated their drug war. We found ourselves the recipients of more than an occasional flyover and were visited five times. During the early years of the drug war, officers were allowed to use their discretion in such situations. At each meeting we were able to explain our position regarding my medical use of marihuana, and each time the officers spared our privacy and some of my stash. We have never considered our actions criminal and have always spoken without reserve when approached by CAMP (Campaign Against Marihuana Production) officers or police. We told them about the debilitating side effects of pharmaceuticals and explained that marihuana offered a reprieve from epileptic seizures and allowed me to live a relatively productive life. On one occasion a CAMP officer let us go after telling us he understood my fate because his father had epilepsy.

Our work with other patients began in 1974, when my grandmother contracted leukemia. She encountered the usual barrage of chemotherapies, and we stood by impotently watching while this powerful woman faded before our eyes. Then I suggested that she try marihuana, explaining that it might help with nausea. When I told her I had been using it for seizure control she was impressed, for my family had lived with my illness, too. She tried the marihuana and soon felt hungry; the next morning she said it was the best night's sleep she had ever had. She used marihuana until her life ended in 1976. She was first of more than twenty friends and family members with varying diseases that we provided with marihuana before our first arrest.

With the increase in federal money for marihuana eradication and the introduction of a zero-tolerance policy, the attitudes of the authorities began to change. The fervor of the drug war was clamoring for a new high. In August 1992, CAMP sheriffs arrived at our home with guns drawn. Mike and I were separated, questioned, and arrested, despite our explanations. We had discussed many times our willingness to go to jail if necessary for what we believed, but I was terrified by the prospect of three years in state prison and the possibility that I would no longer have access to marihuana for seizure control. I credit Mike for encouraging me to stand for moral justice in the face of this most unjust law. I used the defense of medical necessity and succeeded—for the first time ever in California.

We thought this victory implied impunity, and the next spring we began to grow more marihuana in our garden. But in September 1993 CAMP sheriffs came again. This time they ravaged our home, searching every inch with the thoroughness of an ant colony. We were infuriated. We felt violated. I had won the case just six months before. Why would they harass us further when the courts had let us go and the district attorney had told the sheriff he would not press charges? During this encounter I told the CAMP officials that for sixteen years we had been distributing marihuana to people dying of cancer and AIDS. These were people we loved who had found great benefit from marihuana. The sheriffs were not impressed and added a charge of distribution to the cultivation charge. The charges are still pending [in 1996].

I decided to seek public support by appealing candidly to the community in a county that had supported a resolution to make marihuana legal for medical use. The response has been overwhelming. I have been appointed to the Alcohol and Drug Abuse Commission, and I have started a patient/caregiver co-operative, which provides marihuana to terminally and chronically ill patients who have a doctor's note. Members of our co-op receive medical marihuana free of charge or for a nominal donation. We educate patients regarding the medical use of marihuana, including cultivation methods. We have recorded the effectiveness of different varieties of marihuana, and we find that different strains affect the symptoms of different ailments. Our goal is to offer a community model that empowers patients and caregivers to provide for themselves and for one another.

Because controlled studies are not yet available, it is impossible to say how many patients with seizure disorders might get relief from cannabis. But we do know from cases like those presented above that some people are helped by cannabis and nothing else. Furthermore, they do not have to pay a high price in toxic or even uncomfortable side effects. Many epileptic patients are unsuccessfully treated with three or more antiepileptic drugs taken simultaneously, a practice that greatly increases the severity of toxic effects. The value of cannabis — for some patients, a unique value — is especially clear when overall quality of life is considered as well as adequacy of seizure control.

MULTIPLE SCLEROSIS

Multiple sclerosis (MS) is a disorder in which patches of myelin (the protective covering of nerve fibers) in the brain and spinal cord are destroyed and the normal functioning of the nerve fibers themselves is interrupted. It seems to be an autoimmune response in which the body's defense system treats the myelin as a foreign invader. The symptoms usually appear in early adulthood, then come and go unpredictably for years. Attacks last weeks to months, and remission is often incomplete, with gradual deterioration and eventual severe disability. Injury, infection, or stress may cause a relapse. The average survival time is thirty years, but some patients deteriorate much faster, and others stabilize after a few attacks.

The symptoms depend on which part of the central nervous system is affected by demyelination. Because the brain and spinal cord control the whole body, the effects may appear almost anywhere. Some common symptoms are tingling, numbness, impaired vision, difficulty in speaking, painful muscle spasms, loss of coordination and balance (ataxia), fatigue, weakness or paralysis, tremors, loss of bladder and/or bowel control, urinary tract infections, constipation, skin ulcerations, and severe depression.

No effective treatment is known. Corticosteroids, especially adrenocorticotropic hormone (ACTH) and prednisone, provide some relief for the acute symptoms, but they also cause weight gain and sometimes mental disturbances. The drugs most commonly used to treat muscle spasms are diazepam (Valium), baclofen (Lioresal), and dantrolene (Dantrium). Diazepam and other drugs in the benzodiazepine class, which must be given in large doses, cause drowsiness and can be addictive. Both dantrolene and baclofen are of marginal medical utility. Baclofen is a sedative and sometimes causes dizziness, weakness, or confusion. Dantrolene is a last resort because of potentially lethal liver damage; it also has a variety of other side effects, including drowsiness, dizziness, weakness, general malaise, abdominal cramps, diarrhea, speech and visual disturbances, seizures, headaches, impotence, tachycardia, erratic blood pressure, clinical depression, myalgia, feelings of suffocation, and confusion. Understandably, many patients cannot tolerate the immediate side effects of the standard drugs or become concerned about the long-term effects.

The use of marihuana in multiple sclerosis is illustrated in this account by Greg Paufler, a thirty-seven-year-old resident of upstate New York:

In 1973 I noticed a feeling of numbness in my left thumb that began to spread to the rest of my left hand. I explained the symptoms to a doctor, who diagnosed my problem as neuritis, said it would clear up in a few days, and recommended vitamin supplements. Within a week the numbness was gone, but I began to have difficulty maintaining my balance and sometimes had trouble walking.

By the early spring of 1974, my health was much worse, although I continued to take my vitamins. My stumbling and falling became an office joke at the insurance company where I worked as a salesman. Other employees would laughingly ask me if I had been drinking. My supervisor complained that I was seeing fewer clients and writing fewer orders. I told him that the numbness in my legs interfered with driving a car and that I was finding it increasingly difficult to write (I did not reveal that I was barely able to write at all). He did not seem satisfied with these explanations. Soon afterward a co-worker and close friend persuaded me to obtain a second opinion. As I walked into the doctor's waiting room, I fell flat on my face and cut my knee. The nurse helped me into the office. I tried to stand on my own and fell again. I told the doctor that I had sharp spasms and numbness in my legs and could not tell where my feet were without looking at them. The doctor, a general practitioner, insisted that I be hospitalized immediately, despite my protests; he said I might have a brain tumor.

I remained in the hospital for seven days of observation and medical tests supervised by a team of physicians headed by a neurologist. During this time I lost all control over my limbs and experienced severe, painful spasms. My arms and legs became numb. I could no longer walk. I was given intravenous injections of ACTH, a powerful steroid, but it didn't help; it only kept me awake and increased my appetite dramatically. On the day of my release, the supervising neurologist told me I was suffering from multiple sclerosis. He said there was no cure, but drugs like ACTH could slow its progress. He then told me to go home and get plenty of rest. He made an appointment to see me in his office—an appointment that, as it turned out, I could not keep because I was too weak to make the trip. Instead the doctor had a nurse come to our home and show my wife how to inject me with ACTH.

Shortly after I returned home, and while I was bedridden, some friends came to visit and we smoked a few marihuana cigarettes. Afterward I felt better, but attributed that effect to the mild "high." My spasms also became less severe, but I gave the daily injections of ACTH credit for that. Despite some improvement, I remained bedridden and soon began to feel the effects of chronic high-dose steroid therapy. I retained fluids and became bloated; I gained a hundred pounds in six weeks because ACTH made me ravenously hungry. I had sleepless nights. I started losing my concentration. My mental attitude was dismal and I became depressed. After three months of intensive therapy, my condition had barely improved. I could walk only when supported by my wife and a cane or walker.

The doctor told me I had to take ACTH for another three

months, but he was obviously concerned about the side effects. He warned me of the danger of a sudden heart attack or respiratory failure. To reduce fluid retention, he prescribed a powerful diuretic which he acknowledged could cause kidney stones or death from kidney failure. The steroid therapy was still not working, and its adverse effects became worse. My weight rose from 170 pounds before taking ACTH to 300 pounds within several weeks after starting the second round of ACTH therapy. Breathing became difficult as fluids pressed against my lungs. My feet and legs were swollen. None of my clothes fit. I developed severe, intense depression marked by abrupt mood shifts. I would become profoundly upset for no reason; I would suddenly start to cry or have violent thoughts. After six months I felt that I had lost all control over my life. On rare, very good days I could shuffle across my bedroom by leaning against the wall and using my wife and a walker for support. Even then I could not maintain my balance or support my weight, and I often fell. Most of the time I was bedridden. My spasms continued, and my limbs were out of control.

At the end of the sixth month I saw my doctor again and told him my condition was getting worse. He said that my MS was very severe and had progressed very rapidly; only ACTH could help. He recommended another three months and increased the dose by 50 percent. He also prescribed a sleeping pill and Valium to reduce my spasms. I agreed to give ACTH another try, but changed my mind a couple of days later. I could not take it any longer. If the only choice was MS or this treatment, I would rather have the MS. When I stopped taking ACTH, my vision became blurred and I had episodes of tunnel vision. I could not focus and lost my ability to read; the MS was attacking me in an entirely different way. My doctor became very worried and immediately prescribed prednisone, a powerful oral steroid. Again I received little therapeutic benefit but there were many adverse effects, this time even more intense; in less than a month I gained more than eighty pounds. But there was worse to come. Although I did not know it, the steroids were stripping my body of critically important potassium.

One day, while sitting in my living room, I realized I could not talk. I was semicatatonic. One of my children walked up and spoke to me. I heard her but could not see her and could not respond, except by crying. My wife and daughter immediately took me to a hospital emergency room. I have no memory of the trip and did not know where I was when we arrived. I remember being slumped in a chair alone, then surrounded by nearly a dozen doctors and nurses, all frantically talking. They asked me questions I am not sure I heard. When I tried to respond I could not speak. Medical records indicate that I nearly died that day; my body had almost no potassium in it. I was given massive injections and an oral potassium supplement.

This experience caused me to become deeply disenchanted with drugs, doctors, and hospitals. I stopped taking all steroids, although I continued to use Valium and other mood-altering drugs. Unable to walk, read, or be with my family, I began smoking marihuana to relieve the boredom, four to six joints a day. One evening some old friends came to visit and we smoked several joints. When they rose to leave I stood up to say good-bye. Everyone in the room suddenly stopped talking and stared at me. I realized that I had spontaneously stood unassisted, as if it were perfectly natural.

I was stunned. My wife and our friends were stunned. I took a few unassisted steps before my legs, weak from atrophy, gave out. I had walked! I wondered if it was the marihuana, and asked my doctor, who dismissed the idea and insisted that marihuana had no beneficial effect on MS. My wife, too, was skeptical, but I kept on experimenting. I soon discovered that when I did not smoke marihuana my spasms were more frequent and intense. When I smoked it, my condition stabilized, then dramatically improved. I could walk unaided, and my vision was less blurred. But my doctor and my wife remained skeptical. In what I now realize was a foolish attempt to prove to others what I already knew to be true, I decided to stop smoking marihuana for six months.

As soon as I stopped I began to lose what I had gained. I had severe spasms in my back muscles. After four months I had lost control of my hands, arms, feet, and legs. My dose of Valium rose to 120 mg daily, and I began to realize that I was chemically dependent, an addict. I stopped taking Valium and suffered a severe withdrawal reaction from this "safe," "medically accepted" drug. I lost all interest in life; I was sleepless, restless, and constantly agitated; I fell into a dark depression; my mood shifts became even more erratic and pronounced; my spasms became intensely painful.

When I could no longer sit up, much less walk, I resumed smoking marihuana daily. Within a few weeks I was able to walk again unaided. I was soon walking half a block alone with some effort. I regained strength as I got more exercise, and my eyesight returned to normal. After six months all my symptoms had improved greatly. The spasms had vanished, and I had regained the ability to read, write, and walk. One evening I went out with my children and, for the first time in two years, showed them how to kick a soccer ball. I could kick a ball! I felt reborn.

But I was still uncertain whether marihuana was responsible. Marihuana was something I used for fun, a social drug. I did not believe that such a simple and safe drug could produce such a startling improvement. It was all the easier to ignore the obvious because my doctor and my wife continued to laugh at the idea. To show myself that it was not really the marihuana that was helping, I decided to stop smoking yet again. At first gradually and then more rapidly, the muscle spasms returned. Within a few weeks I needed a cane, then a walker. Eventually I was bedridden again. After four months I decided to start smoking again. My condition immediately stabilized, then began to improve. I was happy but very confused. This pattern continued. I would smoke marihuana until my condition improved, then stop. For reasons I cannot explain, I found it hard to believe that marihuana was really the cause of these dramatic changes in my health.

In 1980 my brother showed me a newspaper article about an MS patient in Washington named Sam Diana who had convinced a court of law that his use of marihuana was a "medical necessity." I was astonished to learn that I was not the only MS patient getting relief from marihuana. It was even more astonishing that doctors, researchers, and other MS patients had supported Mr. Diana's claim and the court had ruled in his favor. I no longer felt the need to prove to myself or anyone else that marihuana was helpful; I started listening to my body and went back to smoking regularly.

For the past seven years my MS has been well controlled, except when I run out of marihuana and cannot find or afford more. Most MS patients grow progressively weaker and more crippled; I have improved. I can stand on one foot with my eyes closed. I walk completely unaided. I can actually run! This may seem insignificant to someone who has never been bedridden, crippled, and unable to move or speak, but to me it is a miracle. On top of all that, marihuana allows me to maintain an erection long enough to complete the sex act. I have never become chemically dependent on marihuana, and I have no withdrawal symptoms when I stop smoking. Compared to the steroids, tranquilizers, and sedatives usually prescribed for MS patients, marihuana is remarkably safe and benign.

My doctor is amazed by the improvement in my symptoms. On a scale of one to 100, he rates my physical and mental health at 95. He no longer insists that marihuana is useless. At the end of our last meeting he looked me in the eye and told me to keep doing whatever it is I am doing, because it works.

I do not like breaking the law. I do not enjoy paying terribly inflated prices to drug dealers for an unregulated, uncontrolled product. But I do like to walk, talk, read, write, and see. My doctor and I are now exploring the possibility of gaining legal access to marihuana through the Food and Drug Administration's Compassionate IND program, despite the extraordinarily slow and complicated procedure required.[17]

17. Paufler never received a Compassionate IND; the program was discontinued shortly after he wrote this account.

Most MS patients in the United States now learn about marihuana through support groups or the grapevine. Many anecdotes testify to its capacity to relieve tremors and loss of muscle coordination. Neurologists often hear about it from their patients. Yet the medical literature includes only a few cases like the following one, reported in 1983:

A 30-year-old man had a ten-year history of MS consisting of exacerbations and remissions, resulting in paraparesis, diplopia, ataxia, numbness and parasthesia in all extremities, urinary retention, incontinence, and impotence. Medical treatments had included ACTH, corticosteroids, and Imuran [azathioprine, an immunosuppressive agent]. A disabling tremor had been a consistent problem for more than a year. The tremor was maximal in the head and neck and resulted in particular problems while eating, because it increased as efforts were made to put food in the mouth. The tremor was diminished, but not abolished, when the patient was supine with his head fully supported. It disappeared with sleep. Treatment with diazepam, alcohol, propranolol, and physostigmine were uniformly unsuccessful. Marihuana had been used to control the tremor on an almost daily basis for at least one year prior to this study without evidence of diminishing response. The initial 5 mg dose of THC resulted in a decrease in head and neck tremor within 30 to 60 minutes which lasted approximately six hours. The dose resulted in a very mild "high" which did not appear to impair judgment. Mild hand ataxia seen in finger-nose-finger testing was little changed, but the patient's ability to write was considerably improved [fig. 2], and his use of eating utensils was markedly improved. When placebo capsules were substituted no improvement occurred in spite of a "high" sensation. Repeated testing with the active drug on two occasions again demonstrated the response.[18]

In another report, neurologists at the University of Göttingen, Germany, noticed that one of their patients, a thirty-year-old man with

18. D. B. Clifford, "Tetrahydrocannabinol for Tremor in Multiple Sclerosis," *Annals of Neurology* 13 (1983): 669–671.

CONTROL   THC 5 MG

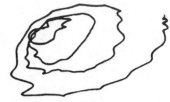   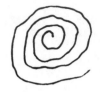

TREMOR RECORDING-HEAD

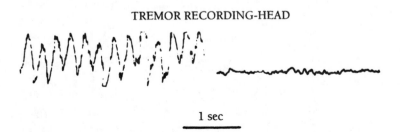

1 sec

Figure 2. Handwriting sample and movement artifact from head, recorded before and 90 minutes after ingestion of 5 mg of tetrahydrocannabinol. Reproduced from D. B. Clifford, "Tetrahydrocannabinol for tremor in multiple sclerosis," Annals of Neurology 13:6 (1983): 669–671.

multiple sclerosis, smoked marihuana to treat his motor and sexual handicaps. They tested him with clinical ratings, electromyographic study of his leg reflexes, and electromagnetic recording of his hand tremors (fig. 3). Their conclusion was that cannabis warranted further evaluation as a treatment for both muscle spasms and ataxia (loss of

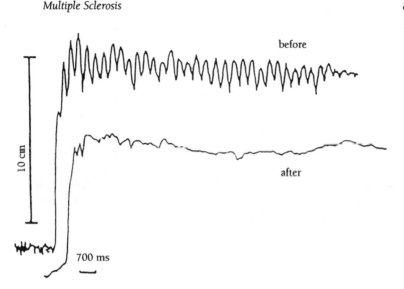

Figure 3. Electromagnetic recording of the finger and hand action tremor in a pointing task the morning before and the evening after smoking a marihuana cigarette. Reproduced from H. M. Meinck, P. W. Schonle, and B. Conrad, "Effect of cannabinoids on spasticity and ataxia in multiple sclerosis," Journal of Neurology 236 (1989): 120–122.

coordination).[19] These cases suggesting that marihuana provides relief for both tremors and ataxia are of special interest, because no drug now legally available has both these effects.

Debbi Talshir is a forty-three-year-old divorced woman who has treated her multiple sclerosis with cannabis for seventeen years. She tells her story:

I was diagnosed with multiple sclerosis in 1977. One of its first symptoms was optic neuropathy. The optic nerve connects the brain and eye, and optic neuropathy is a degeneration of that connection. It can cause partial blindness. First a big cloud ap-

19. H. M. Meinck, P. W. Schönle, and B. Conrad, "Effect of Cannabinoids on Spasticity and Ataxia in Multiple Sclerosis," *Journal of Neurology* 236 (1989): 120–122.

peared in my vision and I could not see so well; the cloud then
became black in the right eye.

For the neuropathy I was given ACTH. I gained about 100
pounds because I retained water and my appetite increased dramatically (I was always starving). The ACTH also caused mood
swings that made me intolerable to my co-workers and friends.
Even I was frightened by them. Finally they subsided, only to
return a year and a half later, along with the optic neuropathy.
This time a co-worker recommended marihuana and I smoked a
couple of cigarettes. I didn't gain weight or have mood swings,
and the optic neuropathy subsided in three weeks.

As the MS progressed, I was given Lioresal [baclofen] for
muscle spasms. Yes, it caused side effects: drowsiness and just
general lethargy. I found that marihuana stopped the spasms and
relaxed my muscles, but not so much that they became useless. My neurologist at Massachusetts General Hospital, where I
was first diagnosed, and my current neurologist here on Cape
Cod know that I use marihuana to manage those symptoms
and others. It is on my record, but they won't [cannot] supply
legal prescriptions—very disheartening, but understandable in
the present climate of the drug war. Since 1980 I have been confined to a wheelchair. I cannot eat unless I smoke some marihuana first; it relaxes the sphincter muscles in my stomach and
esophagus. My loss of appetite is profound, but if I smoke a marihuana cigarette I am relaxed and can hold food down. Often I
have difficulty breathing. I don't understand why smoking anything would relax the breathing mechanisms, but marihuana
does.

To me, marihuana is essential. I don't shake any more, I can
eat, I can breathe. It even has a very good effect on my neuro-
genic bladder—a neurological disorder in which a person loses
control of the sphincter muscles of the bladder. If there is even a
drop of urine in the bladder, the sphincter muscles go into spasm
and you lose urine. Marihuana doesn't cure it, but it helps. I generally smoke five marihuana cigarettes a day.

I am very angry that I have to deal with people whom I wouldn't ordinarily socialize with, such as drug dealers. I also have to save my pennies if I am going to get any marihuana, and it is getting increasingly difficult to find. I find myself running around, making phone calls, and spending most of my time looking for it.

Talshir notes that cannabis helps her to control her bladder, a problem for up to 90 percent of patients with multiple sclerosis. Sometimes cannabis enables them to lead normal lives after years of being housebound by fear of embarrassment. Three women with multiple sclerosis have told us that although they began using cannabis for the relief of muscle spasms, they found it equally helpful for bladder control. One says she would use it for that reason alone if necessary.

Cannabis may also be helpful for loss of bowel control in multiple sclerosis. A forty-year-old man troubled by this symptom told us:

> Though at first skeptical of the weed I had smoked occasionally since college, I now consider cannabis use an effective counter to many MS symptoms. Along with its anti-spasticity and anti-depressant effects, cannabis ensures "regularity" of defecation as its most dramatic benefit. I start to poop in my pants within two to three days unless I smoke my daily dose of one cigarette. Believe me, this means a great deal in the struggle to maintain a positive self-image. Though clearly not an MS cure, regular marihuana use, for me, provides "regularity" as the most dramatic among other benefits.

A patient whose loss of muscle coordination proved to be an early symptom of multiple sclerosis was brought to our attention by her psychiatrist. For several years he had been trying to get her to give up the habit of smoking a small amount of marihuana at bedtime to defeat her chronic insomnia. After persuading her to stop, he sought advice from us when he realized that the cannabis had been suppressing the symptoms of her previously undiagnosed multiple sclerosis; ataxia appeared when she stopped smoking and disappeared when she started again. He was concerned because he thought marihuana was highly toxic; our assurances that it was not relieved that fear. His patient tells her story:

> I had finally gotten where I wanted to be. What I lacked in education I had made up for with hard work, long hours, and the boss that every young businesswoman dreams of. Starting at twenty-one as the lowest paid clerk in a small local company, I was now, at forty-five, a finance executive for a billion-dollar electronics firm.
>
> The work was hard, fast, and demanding, but very satisfying. Stepping the pace down at the end of the day was difficult, and I found that smoking a very small amount of marihuana at bedtime allowed me to relax and get to sleep. By 1986 I had been smoking for about fifteen years and wasn't concerned that such a small amount could be harmful.
>
> From 1986 through 1989 I fought a continuing low-key battle with my psychiatrist about this. I felt that my experience was entirely positive and that any ill effects would have become evident in fifteen years. My doctor, however, thought I should not use an untested and, incidentally, illegal drug.
>
> In October 1989 I agreed to replace marihuana with Desyrel [trazodone, an antidepressant with sedative properties]. Although it was not as effective, and I had hangovers the morning after, the substitution seemed acceptable for a few days. On the sixth morning, however, I realized that I had lost most of my ability to balance. I could barely stand upright or walk without support. While driving to the doctor's office, I also found that what I call my autopilot had been wiped clean. Activities normally performed subconsciously, like driving, now required conscious thought. I even had to relearn the way the key turned to unlock the car. I was also more tired than I had ever been before.
>
> In the next six weeks I took no drugs at all, not even an aspirin, while doctors tested me for every disease known to Western medicine. During this time my symptoms did not improve. After the tests I received the devastating news that I had multiple sclerosis, an incurable nerve disease with little hope of mean-

ingful treatment. Although I had been told that MS symptoms come and go without warning, I was disturbed by the apparent coincidence and hesitantly raised the marihuana question with a neurologist. I was given an angry lecture and instructions to return only when I could pass a drug screening test.

I couldn't let it go at that. Logic dictated that I at least try smoking marihuana. My doctor [psychiatrist] was still opposed, but did express some interest in what might happen, so I decided to start. About a week later I noticed an improvement, and a few weeks later I was able to return to work at about 85 percent of normal.

The improvement could have been spontaneous—MS is very capricious—but I wasn't about to take a chance, and I went on smoking until the spring of 1990, when I ran out of marihuana and was unable to get any more. A week later all my symptoms were again severe.

My doctors still thought it was a coincidence, but I didn't. I began a nationwide search for supplies of marihuana and for a neurologist who would at least listen to my story with an open mind. I found the marihuana, but not the neurologist. Since it is illegal to conduct experiments with marihuana, there is no scientific evidence of its value; and, because there is no scientific evidence of its value, the government will not allow experimentation.

When I finally received some marihuana from a friend and resumed smoking, I only returned to 60 percent of normal and could work only at home. Later in 1990 the entire sequence was repeated, and this time I returned to less than 50 percent of normal. I could no longer work more than a half hour at a time. Early in 1991 I was retired at 100 percent disability.

I still have a small supply of marihuana and am afraid of what will happen when it runs out. In the meantime I am praying that the laws can be changed.

There are hints in this case and others that cannabis not only relieves the symptoms of multiple sclerosis—muscle spasms, tremor, loss of muscle coordination (ataxia) and bladder control, insomnia—but also retards the progression of the disease. Multiple sclerosis is a disorder caused by an immune system gone haywire; current treatments include the use of steroids that suppress immune functioning. Although smoked marihuana apparently does not increase susceptibility to infectious disease, there is evidence that THC has immunosuppressive effects. With this in mind, a group of investigators tested its ability to suppress experimental autoimmune encephalitis (EAE), a disease that has been used as a laboratory model of multiple sclerosis in guinea pigs. When animals were exposed to the disease and then treated with placebo, all developed severe EAE and more than 98 percent died. Animals treated with delta-9-THC had either mild symptoms or none; more than 95 percent survived, and on inspection their brain tissue was much less inflamed.[20] In a subsequent study, delta-8-THC (a less psychoactive analog of delta-9-THC) was administered for up to twenty-one days to two strains of rats inoculated for EAE. It significantly reduced neurological deficits in both strains.[21]

PARAPLEGIA AND QUADRIPLEGIA

Paraplegia is weakness or paralysis of muscles in the lower body caused by disease or injury in the middle or lower part of the spinal cord. If the injury is near the neck, the arms as well as the legs are affected, and quadriplegia develops. Paraplegia and quadriplegia are often accompanied by pain and muscle spasms; standard treatments are opioids for the pain, and baclofen and diazepam for the muscle spasms. Many paraplegics and quadriplegics have now discovered that cannabis not only relieves their pain more safely than opioids but also effectively suppresses their muscle jerks and tremors. The following account by Chris Woiderski is illustrative:

    20. W. D. Lyman, J. R. Sonett, C. F. Brosnan, R. Elkin, and M. B. Bornstein, "Delta-9-tetrahydrocannabinol: A Novel Treatment for Experimental Autoimmune Encephalitis," *Journal of Neuroimmunology* 23 (1989): 73–81.
    21. I. Wirguin, R. Mechoulam, A. Breuer, E. Schezen, J. Weidenfeld, and T. Brenner, "Suppression of Experimental Autoimmune Encephalomyelitis by Cannabinoids," *Immunopharmacology* 28:3 (November–December 1994): 209–214.

In June 1989, I was twenty-seven years old and had been working as an industrial engineer for five and a half years, selling pneumatic and automation equipment to manufacturing plants and factories. I was pretty successful at it. I had used marihuana off and on for several years to relax. After a long hard day I would go home, have dinner with my girlfriend, smoke some marihuana, and unwind. I usually spent evenings in my home office, and I found that smoking marihuana not only relaxed me but helped me concentrate on my work.

I would sometimes think that things just couldn't get any better for me. I had a good job, made excellent money, and lived with the woman I was going to marry in a few months. Then, in June 1989, I suffered an accidental gunshot wound. I was rushed to a hospital and wheeled into surgery. I awoke the next evening in a semi-coherent state, feeling the pain from tubes in my chest and throat. After ten days in the intensive care unit, a neurologist told me there was nothing he could do for me. Although the bullet had missed my spinal cord, swelling had left me permanently paralyzed from the chest down. When I finally realized I would never be cured, I got angry, and the anger never went away.

I was no longer able to work, so I subsisted on a meager Social Security pension. Luckily, I had served in the Navy and was eligible to receive medical supplies and care from the Veterans' Administration. After two months of watching me try to do the simplest tasks (dressing, showering, getting in and out of bed), my girlfriend just couldn't take it any more and moved back to her parents' house.

Four months after my injury I began to experience the strange and somewhat painful sensations known as muscle spasms. At first they affected only my feet and lower legs, but soon I had them in all my paralyzed muscles. I was given a drug called baclofen, but even the maximum dosage did not provide much relief. There were plenty of unpleasant side effects, though— drowsiness, severe headaches, excessive sweating, insomnia, and dry mouth.

My spasms became more and more violent. After they caused

me to fall out of bed, the doctors added 20 mg a day of Valium, then another 20 mg. I was becoming a pharmacological zombie. There were many other paralyzed patients at the VA hospital. Some had been paraplegics for more than twenty years. They told me they had thrown away their prescription spasm medications years ago and now used marihuana instead. They said it worked better and had far fewer side effects. I tried it. One marihuana cigarette gave me immediate relief without the debilitating side effects of Valium and baclofen. Everyday tasks like showering and dressing became remarkably easier to accomplish. Since then, whenever I can find marihuana, I smoke three to four cigarettes a day. I have few or no spasms, and I am spared the need to take twelve very toxic and addictive pills daily. I have also discovered that I can achieve an erection when I smoke marihuana; the only way I could do that before was by injecting prostaglandin directly into my penis.

About two-thirds of the paralyzed patients I've met use marihuana to control muscle spasms and pain. Present Drug Enforcement Administration regulations forbid our doctors to prescribe marihuana for us. The government is now waging a war on drugs that in effect targets me and other paralyzed patients. This is not only unreasonable and unfair, but blatantly immoral. Because we choose to use the most effective and safest drug for our condition, the government unjustly puts us in the same criminal category as heroin junkies.

Woiderski notes that marihuana enabled him to achieve a normal erection. One report in the medical literature confirms this effect. A thirty-year-old patient had suffered from MS for six years and was wheelchair-bound because of muscle spasms and ataxia. His erections lasted less than five minutes, and he was unable to ejaculate. When he smoked marihuana, both his motor functions and his sexual functions improved immediately. He can now sustain an erection for more than half an hour, and his sexual life is satisfactory.[22]

22. H. M. Meinck, P. W. Schönle, and B. Conrad, "Effect of Cannabinoids on Spasticity and Ataxia in Multiple Sclerosis," *Journal of Neurology* 236 (1989): 120–122.

Russ Hokanson is a fifty-three-year-old paraplegic man who has been using cannabis as an analgesic for three decades, ever since he discovered that it gave him the best relief for severe pain following an accident:

In April 1965 I was in an automobile accident. The car rolled over several times, catching me between the door and roof and nearly cutting me in half. I suffered a crushed lower spine, a burst spleen, broken ribs, punctured lungs, a broken leg, and mutilated intestines. I nearly died on the spot. The doctors at the hospital told my father not to bother driving the 900 miles to see me, because I would not make it through the night. Nevertheless, he did come (a high-speed drive with police escort), and I surprised the doctors by staying alive.

When I regained consciousness I was strapped in a bed with tubes inserted in both legs and both arms, down my nose and down my throat, and through my penis into my bladder. I was in extreme pain and drifted in and out of consciousness. It took two months for my condition to stabilize. They removed my spleen, set my broken leg, and performed three major reconstructive surgeries on my back, including spinal fusion—using parts of my hip bone to reconstruct my spine, which had been shattered into small pieces. I also needed two laminectomies to take the pressure off my spinal cord.

I was in the hospital for about a year and saw several people die next to me. Once I was put in a rotating bed but not properly strapped in; I fell on the floor and broke my leg again. Now it is one and one-half inches shorter than the other leg. I had a bed sore the size of a large dinner plate over my buttocks, exposing the pelvic bones, and needed a large skin graft to heal it. I also had open ulcerated sores on my legs and feet, one of which lasted four years and recurred as late as 1976. During one operation my catheter became tangled in my bed frame and pulled out; I woke up in a pool of urine and blood. In another operation I was given the wrong blood type and nearly died—I had huge welts all over my body, my tongue swelled up, and I couldn't breathe.

All through the hospital stay I was in severe pain. I could never sleep more than one and a half hours at a time, and then only when I was totally exhausted. Only large doses of Demerol [a morphine derivative] could ease the pain for a few hours. I got hooked on Demerol and went through a withdrawal reaction when I quit taking it.

After nearly a year in the hospital I decided I couldn't spend the rest of my life there and had to take control of my destiny, so I signed myself out—against the wishes of my doctors, who thought I wouldn't survive on the outside. At that time I couldn't even put on my socks and shoes, but I was determined to care for myself somehow.

Before the accident I had had two years of college, and I wanted to finish. I somehow managed to return and attend classes, taking several Darvon pain pills every 1½ hours. College was where I first smoked marihuana, and I found it had many desirable effects. Most important, it not only relieved my chronic pain but allowed me to rise above it by reducing the anxiety—that sick feeling in the pit of the stomach that accompanies pain. I am subject to stabbing pains in otherwise paralyzed and numb parts of my body. They are hard to control with standard pain medicine, but marihuana helps. Besides, pain relief from standard narcotics tends to diminish over time, so that you need more and more pills. With marihuana it is the other way around—I need less for the same effect as time goes on.

Marihuana is also a good sedative; it allows me to sleep longer without waking up in pain. It is a great antidepressant that helps me to accept my disability and develop a positive outlook on life. That has been a major hurdle for me, since I used to be athletic—a mountain climber, skier, and member of the college wrestling team. Marihuana also stimulates my appetite and helps me overcome the disinterest in food caused by chronic pain. It even helped me restore bladder control. When I left the hospital, I quit using a catheter and urine bag and instead relied on diapers and paper towels stuck in my underwear. I found that when

I smoked marihuana I could feel my penis and bladder control muscles better and know when I was about to "leak"; marihuana also seemed to tone my sphincter muscle, so that I "leaked" less, and eventually achieved normal urine control. Marihuana gave me back a normal sex life by allowing me to achieve an erection and feel sensations in my penis.

As my interest in life grew, so did my ability to concentrate on intellectual work and my desire to lead a natural lifestyle. I read all I could on health. After graduating from Kalamazoo College with a science teaching degree in botany and biology, I was awarded a fellowship for a master's degree in horticulture and plant science from the University of Delaware. I became a vegetarian and regained a keen interest in religion—seeking to treat all things with respect and to experience God in my life and love in my heart. I learned how to grow my food organically and how to nurture the land and soil around me through natural methods such as composting, soil remineralization, earthworms, and seaweed nutrition.

For twenty-five years I have had no health insurance; I prefer to depend on my own resources, including natural farming and natural medicine. This led me to the inevitable conclusion that I should start growing my own medicine. As a result, on August 10, 1993, I was arrested. I am now facing a felony trial with a possible jail sentence, and the State of New Hampshire is trying to seize my house and land. It seems incredible that this could be the result of growing my own medicine, and even more incredible that I am charged with criminal intent when my only intent was to heal myself.

Hokanson's case was eventually settled with the payment of a fine. He is technically on probation but does not expect to be further troubled by the authorities.

Once again, many patients have discovered through word of mouth or support groups a medical use of marihuana that doctors are not supposed to tell them about. The odor of marihuana smoke is said to be omnipresent on some VA hospital paraplegia and quadriplegia wards. A survey of forty-three persons with spinal cord injuries conducted in 1982 indicated that twenty-two of them were using marihuana for muscle spasms.[23] The percentage has probably increased in the past decade. Yet, again, very little on the subject appears in the medical literature. We have been able to find only one recent study.

In 1990 three Swiss neurologists reported on the treatment of a paraplegic patient with painful spasms in both legs who was being constantly medicated with baclofen (Lioresal), clonazepam (Klonopin, an antianxiety drug related to Valium), and codeine for pain. The experiment took place in two stages. In the first stage the patient took oral THC instead of codeine fourteen times over a period of three months. In the second phase he was given either 5 mg of oral THC, 50 mg of oral codeine, or a placebo. The three experimental conditions were each applied eighteen times in the course of five months. He continued to take baclofen and clonazepam throughout the experiment. As compared with placebo, both codeine and THC improved the quality of sleep. Both produced an analgesic effect, but only THC reduced muscle spasms. Both THC and codeine also improved the patient's bladder control, mood, and ability to concentrate on intellectual work. Because THC was as good as codeine in most respects and better at preventing muscle spasms, the neurologists concluded that it should be considered in the treatment of paraplegics.[24]

AIDS

The American AIDS epidemic first came to notice in 1981, when five homosexual men in Los Angeles were found to have developed a mysterious and profound immune deficiency that was being exploited by opportunistic infections (microorganisms that are normally harmless but become dangerous when the immune system is impaired). In

23. J. Malec, R. F. Harvey, and J. J. Cayner, "Cannabis Effect on Spasticity in Spinal Cord Injury," *Archives of Physical and Medical Rehabilitation* 63 (March 1982): 116–118.

24. M. Maurer, V. Henn, A. Dittrich, and A. Hofmann, "Delta-9-tetrahydrocannabinol Shows Antispastic and Analgesic Effects in a Single Case Double-blind Trial," *European Archives of Psychiatry and Clinical Neuroscience* 240 (1990): 104.

1984 the human immunodeficiency virus (HIV) was found to be the cause of AIDS. By now more than 311,000 Americans have died of the disease; nearly one million are infected with the virus, and perhaps as many as half a million are ill. Although the spread of AIDS has slowed among homosexuals, the reservoir is so huge that the number of cases is sure to grow. Women and children as well as both heterosexual and homosexual men are now being affected; the disease is spreading most rapidly among intravenous drug abusers and their sexual partners.

The period of incubation (between infection and the development of symptoms) is variable but averages eight to ten years. It appears that almost all infected persons will eventually become ill. No cure is known. Opportunistic infections and neoplasms (cancerous growths) can be treated in standard ways, and the virus itself can be attacked with antiviral drugs, of which the best known is zidovudine (AZT). Unfortunately, AZT suppresses the production of red blood cells by the bone marrow, decreases the number of white blood cells, and has many damaging effects on the digestive system. It sometimes causes severe nausea, which heightens the danger of semi-starvation for patients who are already suffering from nausea and losing weight because of the illness.

Patients with AIDS need to maintain their appetite and body weight because they may be in danger of wasting away. Furthermore, a good appetite greatly improves their quality of life. Recreational users know that marihuana is an appetite stimulant; it not only makes them hungrier but enhances the flavor of food and the pleasure of eating. This effect has been demonstrated experimentally more than once. In a 1971 study, four groups of subjects received either marihuana extract, alcohol, dextroamphetamine, or a placebo after fasting for twelve hours. Then they were periodically offered milkshakes and asked to say how hungry they were and how much they enjoyed the food. The subjects who took marihuana felt hungrier and ate more; those who took dextroamphetamine felt less hungry and ate less; the effect of alcohol was negligible.[25]

25. L. E. Hollister, "Hunger and Appetite after Single Doses of Marihuana, Alcohol, and Dextroamphetamine," *Clinical Pharmacology and Therapeutics* 12 (January–February 1971): 44–49.

In a later study the body weight and caloric intake of twenty-seven marihuana users and ten control subjects were compared for twenty-one days on a hospital research ward. The marihuana smokers ate more than the controls and gained weight; the controls did not. When they stopped smoking marihuana, they immediately started to eat less.[26] Marihuana's power to enhance appetite was demonstrated again in a 1986 study. Nine subjects smoked two to three placebo cigarettes daily and then switched to marihuana cigarettes of average potency. Their food intake significantly increased, mainly because of extra snacking rather than larger meals.[27]

AIDS wasting syndrome, a common and often fatal outcome of HIV infection, is defined as a loss of 10 percent of body weight or more for unexplained reasons. The FDA has approved only two drugs for its treatment. Megace (megestrol acetate) is a hormone often used to regulate the menstrual cycle, to treat endometriosis (a disorder of the uterine lining), or to stimulate appetite. It is only moderately effective in AIDS patients, and has a number of serious side effects, especially after chronic use.

The other approved drug is Marinol (dronabinol). In the earliest study 70 percent of patients taking it gained weight.[28] In a subsequent study dronabinol effects were evaluated in 139 patients with AIDS-related appetite loss and weight loss of five pounds or more. They were randomly assigned to receive either a placebo or dronabinol twice daily for six weeks. In those who took dronabinol, nausea was decreased and mood and appetite improved. Their weight remained the same on average, and 22 percent gained five pounds or more. Patients taking the placebo lost an average of one pound, and

26. I. Greenberg, J. Kuehnle, J. H. Mendelson, and J. G. Bernstein, "Effects of Marihuana Use of Body Weight and Caloric Intake in Humans," *Journal of Psychopharmacology* (Berlin) 49 (1976): 79–84.

27. R. W. Foltin, J. V. Brady, and M. W. Fischman, "Behavioral Analysis of Marijuana Effects on Food Intake in Humans," *Pharmacology, Biochemistry and Behavior* 25 (1986): 577–582.

28. T. F. Plasse, R. W. Gorter, S. H. Krasnow, et al., "Recent Clinical Experience with Dronabinol," *Pharmacology, Biochemistry and Behavior* 40 (1991): 695–700.

only 10 percent gained five pounds or more. Side effects of dronabinol were mild to moderate. The investigators concluded that it was a safe and effective treatment for appetite loss associated with weight loss in people suffering from AIDS.[29] But many find the effects of dronabinol unpleasant (in the earliest study 20 percent dropped out), and most prefer to smoke cannabis when it is available.

Cannabis has become increasingly popular as a treatment not only for nausea, vomiting, and weight loss but for other AIDS symptoms. Some of the reasons are indicated in the following account by Ron Mason, age thirty-three:

October 19, 1983, was the day I found out I had hepatitis B. For some time I had been noticing a full-page ad in *Gay Chicago* magazine, but I avoided reading it because it looked too depressing (it was a picture of a man in a hospital bed being fed intravenously). When I finally broke down and read it, I found that it was an open letter to the gay community from the Liver Foundation in New Jersey. It said that two-thirds of gay men, whether they knew it or not, were contracting hepatitis B (this was back before "safe sex") at one time or another. Fifty percent of people who are infected with the virus have symptoms, some mild, some severe. Ninety percent develop antibodies after an infection and are no longer susceptible; 10 percent become carriers, and 2 percent die. A vaccine was available, the ad said. So the next time I was at the gay VD clinic, I asked the clerk to screen me for antibodies. It turned out that I had the infection itself. It was too late for vaccination. Now I knew why I was nauseous, often threw up, and tired so easily. Although I lacked appetite, the doctor told me I had to eat. Since I had a liver disease, I naturally gave up drinking (I had never drunk much anyway) and now began to smoke more marihuana. I noticed that my appetite increased dramatically after smoking. I began to smoke daily and gained

29. J. E. Beal, R. Olson, L. Laubenstein, et al., "Dronabinol as a Treatment for Anorexia Associated with Weight Loss in Patients with AIDS," *Journal of Pain and Symptom Management* 10:2 (February 1995): 89–97.

weight rapidly. Two years later I had not yet produced antibodies and was officially designated a hepatitis carrier.

December 23, 1986, is a day I will remember the rest of my life, the day I took the HIV test and found that I had the virus. The huge purplish red marks on my legs, I was to learn, resulted from internal bleeding caused by HIV infection. HIV was also the cause of my severe psoriasis.

In April 1984 I was referred by doctors at a gay VD clinic to what was later to become known as the AIDS clinic in Chicago. I saw doctors there for seven years and gained forty pounds, achieving normal weight. The doctors knew I smoked marihuana and did not forbid it, although they urged moderation. I cannot tolerate AZT because of anemia. All the other antiviral drugs are damaging to my hepatitis-infected liver.

Three years ago one of my doctors told me that I am one of a handful of people who have been going to the clinic for several years and are not dead or gravely ill; the doctors don't know why. I attribute part of my success to smoking marihuana. It makes me feel as if I am living with AIDS rather than just existing. My appetite returns, and once I have eaten, I don't feel sick any more. Marihuana improves my state of mind, and that makes me feel better physically.

I have almost died twice from allergic reactions to Compound Q, an extract of the wild Chinese cucumber root that destroys infected immune cells. Compound Q is illegal, but the government chooses to look the other way. Why can't it do the same for marihuana? Both drugs are illegal and both are used to treat AIDS patients. One will get you in trouble, and the other will not. What a joke!

In the spring of 1990, I was arrested in suburban Chicago for possession of marihuana, and my car was impounded. I have not only lost my medicine but find it difficult to travel to the AIDS clinic in downtown Chicago. My appetite is no longer what it used to be; I have lost fourteen pounds, tire more easily, and sometimes become so run down I feel as though I am going to be sick. I am taking Prozac prescribed by a suburban doctor who knows virtually nothing about AIDS or hepatitis B. I am very depressed and have contemplated suicide several times.

I have had to get cash advances totaling three thousand dollars on my credit card to pay legal fees for two court cases. The felony charge has been dismissed, and I am now trying to get my auto back (the federal civil case) so that I can go to the AIDS clinic. My lawyer tells me I may succeed. Even if I do, how can I relieve the nausea and stimulate my appetite so that I feel better? I tried Marinol and it had no effect. What am I supposed to do? Nothing? If the only way I can stay healthy is to smoke marihuana and therefore feel good enough to eat, why can't I? I wish the government would stop being so hypocritical and let me do what I need to do to live the rest of my days as comfortably as possible.

"Dr. Z," a physician with AIDS, began AZT therapy about two years before he wrote the account presented below. The decline of his immune system soon slowed down, but he also began to suffer from severe nausea and diarrhea (eight to twelve stools per day). His doctor prescribed promethazine and prochlorperazine for nausea, and kaolin, diphenoxylate with atropine, loperamide, and ranitidine for diarrhea and a hyperactive gastrointestinal tract. None of these drugs gave adequate relief. Dr. Z then discovered that smoking small amounts of cannabis throughout the day eliminated the nausea entirely and reduced the number of stools to two to three a day, without the use of any other drugs. Cannabis also relieved the severe fatigue that had been interfering with many of his daily activities. His account follows:

Because of the rabid hysteria that has infected the United States in regard to AIDS and the drug war, I have chosen to remain anonymous. I am a physician with AIDS who believes that marihuana is the best single drug to alleviate many of the maladies associated with AIDS. Some preliminary information will place this discussion in proper perspective.

Like many others, I first experimented with marihuana in col-

lege. I enjoyed the experience, but a pre-med student at a respected Ivy League college had little time for such recreation. In
all, I probably smoked less than a dozen times in college. Medical
school, internship, and residency followed without further marihuana use. I then set up a practice in the small town where I still
live, although I am no longer practicing medicine.

About two years ago I was diagnosed with AIDS. My symptoms included fatigue, headaches, severe leg cramps, nausea, and
occasional sweats. AZT did little to improve any of the symptoms
and even made the nausea worse, but it did slow the progress of
the disease. I had a medicine cabinet filled with barbiturates and
narcotics, all potent legal Schedule II drugs, for my pain and discomfort. Although these drugs helped, they often left me even
more fatigued and lethargic. The pills I took for my leg pains
left my intestinal tract tied up in knots. This, coupled with the
nausea caused by AZT, necessitated another pill, an antiemetic.
All in all, between the pills, the pain, and the nausea, it was not
a lifestyle that made me look forward to starting a new day.

I continued "living" this way until I was invited to a party with
friends I had not seen for some time. I was quite reluctant to go,
since I had the usual throbbing headache and leg cramps, but I
felt I needed to socialize. Someone brought out some grass, and
soon I found myself headache-free and with only the mildest of
leg discomfort. I couldn't believe it—pain-free without the side
effects of the narcotics. In fact, I felt better than at any time since
I had been diagnosed. Trust me, I was not in a semi-comatose
state, either. I was no more relaxed than after a couple of socially
acceptable martinis.

Wondering whether there was some real basis to my discovery,
I spoke to other people with AIDS about marihuana. Almost
unanimously, they said it made them feel better. Unfortunately,
given the current U.S. policy, most of them (including myself)
do not want to risk litigation and exposure. It is tragic enough to
face the diagnosis of AIDS, but compounding the problem with

criminal charges would be unbearable. So we must continue to use potent, addictive Schedule II narcotics and barbiturates when an illegal drug would offer better relief.

Recently I visited Amsterdam, a city where marihuana use is condoned. It is not, strictly speaking, legal, but it is not pun ished as a crime. Believe me, I felt as if I had been cured of AIDS. Although I had usually taken eight to twelve pills a day, I took almost none while I was there. I smoked whenever I felt the need, usually when I became nauseous or had leg cramps or headaches—two or three cigarettes a day. I was often free of symptoms most of the day, without having to worry about being arrested. I could be a responsible adult and use the drug when I felt it was necessary, as I used the pills at home. I felt truly alive once again—a rarity when you suffer from AIDS.

Unfortunately, the cure was short-lived. On returning to the United States I had to start using the legal painkillers and anti-emetics again.

Being both a physician and a patient with HIV disease has been a mixed blessing. I have seen many suffer and die and realize that that will probably be my fate as well. But I also know there is a drug, namely marihuana, that relieves at least some of the suffer ing and can make the life of a person with AIDS more produc-tive. It cannot be prescribed, however, in this kinder and gentler America. This is truly unconscionable. At the rate the epidemic is growing, we will all know someone who is or will be afflicted with HIV. Are we such a ruthless society that we will continue to allow this government's "war on drugs" to force those so afflicted either to become criminals or to suffer needlessly?

Because marihuana is illegal, Dr. Z decided to seek a prescription for Marinol. His doctor knew little about it and was reluctant to pre-scribe it for fear of "addiction" and possible "euphoria." Finally, he wrote a prescription for 5 mg a day, half the dose recommended by a representative of the company that manufactures Marinol. It has taken the general public more than ten years to realize how serious the HIV epidemic is. Unfortunately, it may take physicians another ten years to appreciate the options for treatment.

Dr. Z applied to four pharmacies before he found one that would fill the prescription. After a five-day wait, he obtained the prescribed dose. A five-day trial proved unhelpful. He then increased the dose on his own to 5 mg twice a day and noticed some improvement. But he soon went back to using marihuana, despite the potential legal penalties. Smoking allowed him to titrate the dose for a constant blood level, and illegal marihuana relieved his symptoms better than legal Marinol—a fact that is common knowledge among patients who have tried both.

One recent addition to the anti-AIDS armamentarium is a drug called foscarnet (Foscavir). About 20 percent of AIDS patients develop cytomegalovirus retinitis, an infectious disease of the eye that can cause blindness. Foscarnet was developed to treat this disease and also turned out to prolong the lives of AIDS patients.[30] Unfortunately, among other serious side effects, it causes nausea. There is every reason to believe that this nausea is sensitive to cannabis. If so, and if the hopes for foscarnet pan out, there will be yet another compelling reason for people with AIDS to use marihuana.

Although it is unlikely that a cure for AIDS will be found soon, the situation of people suffering from the disease has become more hopeful. Effective treatments are being developed, and the life expectancy of patients is increasing. For example, AZT is more effective in combination with a newer drug, lamivudine, or 3TC. Protease inhibitors, another recent addition to the anti-AIDS armamentarium, may be the most effective medicines yet. Unfortunately, nausea and vomiting are frequent and serious side effects of both 3TC and protease inhibitors. The advent of these new drugs is the result of medical advances that are transforming HIV infection into a chronic condition that must be

30. AIDS Research Group, in collaboration with the AIDS Clinical Trials Group, "Mortality in Patients with the Acquired Immunodeficiency Syndrome Treated with Either Foscarnet or Ganciclovir for Cytomegalovirus Retinitis," *New England Journal of Medicine* 326 (1992): 213–220.

managed to maintain physical well-being and quality of life. Given this situation, there has been concern about the claim that use of marihuana promotes the development of AIDS or accelerates the collapse of the immune system in people with the disorder Two careful studies have now conclusively shown that this claim is unwarranted.[31] The time has clearly come to integrate cannabis into AIDS treatment.[32]

CHRONIC PAIN

Severe chronic pain is usually treated with opioid narcotics and various synthetic analgesics, but these drugs have many limitations. Opioids are addictive and tolerance develops. The most commonly used synthetic analgesics—aspirin, acetaminophen (Tylenol), and nonsteroidal anti-inflammatory drugs (NSAIDs) like ibuprofen—are not addictive, but they are often insufficiently powerful. Furthermore, they have serious toxic side effects, including gastric bleeding or ulcer and, in the long run, a risk of liver or kidney disease. Stomach bleeding and ulcers induced by aspirin and other NSAIDs are the most common serious adverse drug reactions reported in the United States.[33] These drugs may be responsible for as many as 76,000 hospitalizations and more than 7,600 deaths annually. Heavy drinkers (more than six ounces of alcohol a day) are especially sensitive to

31. R. A. Kaslow, W. C. Blackwelder, D. G. Ostrow, et al., "No Evidence for a Role of Alcohol or Other Psychoactive Drugs in Accelerating Immunodeficiency in HIV-1-Positive Individuals," *JAMA* 261 (1989): 3424–3429. M. J. DiFranco, H. W. Sheppard, D. J. Hunter, et al., "The Lack of Association of Marijuana and Other Recreational Drugs with Progression to AIDS in the San Francisco Men's Health Study," *Annals of Epidemiology* 6 (1996): 283–289.

32. Some patients with advanced cancer may also suffer from loss of appetite, and recent research suggests that cannabis is useful for them as well. See K. Nelson, D. Walsh, P. Deeter, and F. Sheehan, "A Phase II Study of Delta-9-tetrahydrocannabinol for Appetite Stimulation in Cancer-associated Anorexia," *Journal of Palliative Care* 10:1 (Spring 1994): 14–18.

33. S. Girkipal, D. R. Ramey, D. Morfeld, H. Shi, H.T. Hatoum, and J. F. Fries, "Gastrointestinal Tract Complications of Nonsteroidal Anti-inflammatory Drug Treatment in Rheumatoid Arthritis," *Archives of Internal Medicine* 156 (July 22, 1996): 1530–1536.

gastrointestinal effects of NSAIDs. Acetaminophen is increasingly pre-scribed instead because it largely spares the digestive tract, but it can cause liver damage or kidney failure when used regularly for long periods. Medical researchers have estimated that patients who take one to three acetaminophen tablets a day for a year or more account for about 8–10 percent of all cases of end-stage renal disease, a con-dition that is fatal without dialysis or a kidney transplant.[34]

Given the limitations of opioids and the nonaddictive synthetic an-algesics, one might have expected pain specialists to take a second look at cannabis, but the medical literature again suggests little re-consideration until 1975, when one of the few modern studies of can-nabis for the relief of pain was conducted at the University of Iowa. Researchers there gave oral THC or placebo at random to hospital-ized cancer patients who were in severe pain. The THC relieved pain for several hours in doses as low as 5–10 mg, and for even longer at 20 mg. At this dose and in this setting, THC proved to be a sedative as well. It had fewer physical side effects than other commonly used analgesics.[35]

In another study conducted in 1975, codeine, THC, and a placebo were compared in thirty-six patients with advanced cancer. Codeine and THC were equally effective, but some patients found the psycho-active effects of THC (20 mg, compared with 120 mg of codeine) to be uncomfortable. It should be noted that none of these patients knew what drug they were receiving; most had never used marihuana and were unprepared for the consciousness alteration. If they had been prepared, they might not have been uncomfortable.[36]

34. T. V. Perneger, P. Whelton, and M. J. Klag, "Risk of Kidney Failure Associated with the Use of Acetaminophen, Aspirin, and Nonsteroidal Antiinflammatory Drugs," *New England Journal of Medicine* 331:25 (Dec. 22, 1994): 1675–1679. P. M. Ronco and A. Flahault, "Drug-induced End-stage Renal Disease," Editorial, *New England Journal of Medicine,* 331:25 (Dec. 22, 1994): 1711–1712.

35. R. Noyes, S. F. Brunk, D. A. Baram, and A. Canter, "Analgesic Effect of Delta-9-tetrahydrocannabinol," *Journal of Clinical Pharmacology* 15 (February–March 1975): 139–143.

36. R. Noyes, S. F. Brunk, D. H. Avery, and A. Canter, "The Analgesic Properties of Delta-9-tetrahydrocannabinol and Codeine," *Clinical Pharmacology and Therapeutics* 18 (1975): 84–89.

In the same year, Canadian investigators studied the analgesic effect of smoking marihuana in normal subjects, half of whom had used cannabis before. Their tolerance for pain caused by pressure on a thumbnail increased significantly after they smoked marihuana, and the analgesic effect was greater in more experienced users.[37]

Cannabis may be especially useful for certain specific types of chronic pain. The following account is by a man suffering from pseudopseudohypoparathyroidism, a hereditary disorder that results from abnormal responses to a hormone secreted by the parathyroid glands. The function of this hormone is to control the level of calcium in the body. When it is deficient or some of the body's tissues respond to it inadequately (hypoparathyroidism), various symptoms may develop, including muscle spasms, seizures, and, in the variant known as pseudopseudohypoparathyroidism, bone spurs that grow into muscle and nerve tissue and cause agonizing pain.

Irvin Rosenfeld is a forty-two-year-old stockbroker from North Lauderhill, Florida. This is his story:

> I enjoyed a normal childhood until the age of ten. Then one day, while playing Little League ball, I threw someone out at first and my arm became paralyzed for a short time. The incident upset my parents, so we went to see our family doctor, who took an X-ray of my arm. The X-ray appeared to show a fracture that had healed, leaving jagged bone fragments. It made no sense; I had never broken my arm. The doctor sent us to an orthopedic surgeon, who was equally confused and referred me to Children's Hospital in Boston. After a long series of tests, physicians there concluded that I was suffering from multiple congenital cartilaginous exostosis—a rare disease in which the bones develop buds or spurs that grow out into surrounding muscle and nerve fibers, or inward into the bone itself.
>
> The doctors at Children's Hospital discovered more than 250 bone tumors in my arms, legs, and pelvis. In this disease each

37. S. L. Milstein, K. MacCannell, G. Karr, and S. Clark, "Marijuana-produced Changes in Pain Tolerance: Experienced and Non-experienced Subjects," *International Pharmacopsychiatry* 10 (1975): 177–182.

tumor can become malignant, but there were so many in my case that they could not all be surgically removed. The rapid, erratic bone growth is intensely painful and may cause crippling injuries. Bone spurs press against nerve bundles, tangle arteries, and prevent smooth-muscle functioning. If the spurs are jagged, they rip muscle tissue and lead to internal bleeding. If they erupt suddenly and grow quickly, they can interfere with normal growth and cause crippling deformities. The only saving grace is that multiple congenital cartilaginous exostosis does not last for life. Once you stop growing, around age seventeen, the bone spurs stop forming and growing. In theory, the disease will subside if you don't bleed to death or become permanently crippled in your teens.

To prevent that, I underwent three operations on my left leg and one on my right wrist between the ages of ten and seventeen. But day-to-day problems persisted, mainly because of hemorrhaging and muscle tears. By the age of twelve I was often unable to walk or function normally. I was forced out of public school in the eighth grade and was provided with top-notch tutors by the state of Virginia through graduation. On some days I could walk, even run, but for long periods of time I could barely move. Pain was constant and often unbearable; by age fourteen I needed powerful narcotics to control it. At nineteen I was taking 300 mg a day of Sopor [methaqualone, a powerful sedative] and very high doses of Dilaudid [hydromorphone, an opioid narcotic]. These drugs reduced the pain, but they also diminished my mental acuity and interfered with my life. I did not become addicted, but I became extremely fatigued and at times "out of it." If I cut back in order to be more clearheaded, the pain returned. All I remember, beyond the pain, was the waiting—waiting until I would stop growing.

At seventeen, body scans and X-rays indicated that my tumors had stopped growing. Despite persistent pain, I felt that I had passed the crisis and my condition would soon stabilize. But then, at twenty, another massive bone spur erupted in my right ankle. My doctors assumed that it was a delayed manifestation of a latent growth, and they removed it. They said it would probably be the last tumor I ever had. Instead it reappeared and grew with amazing speed, until it stretched five inches up my leg and created a bridge of bone that fused my ankle and leg together. Surgery was impossible; the tumor was too large. The doctors decided to amputate my right foot above the ankle.

At this point I questioned my doctors for the first time. It was increasingly clear that my tumors were continuing to grow and new spurs were developing. If I agreed to the surgery what would need to be amputated next? An arm? Part of another leg? I just said no. No amputation. If the rapidly growing tumor turned malignant, so be it. I was too young to become a cripple for the rest of what might be a short life. I decided to live as well as I could and as whole as I could for as long as I could.

When I was twenty-two, another tumor erupted from my pelvic bone and grew into my groin. This one was surgically removed. Meanwhile, I began to look for other opinions on the nature of my disease. I fruitlessly consulted the Mayo Clinic, the University of Virginia Medical College, the National Institutes of Health (NIH), and the National Cancer Institute (NCI). By this time my drug intake was enormous. I was taking 140 Dilaudid tablets, 30 or more Sopors, and dozens of muscle relaxants and other pills each month. I felt burned out and often walked around in an uncomfortable state. It was difficult to function normally; if I took enough to control the pain, I had difficulty concentrating on my work.

The situation made me dislike drugs intensely. In high school I wrote essays against the use of illegal drugs. It amazed me that people who were well would put a drug into their bodies for fun! I took this attitude with me to college in Florida, where most of the people I met smoked marihuana. At first I strongly resisted "experimenting" with marihuana. I was already "experimenting" with more prescription drugs than my body could handle. But peer pressure works, and I began to smoke marihuana at parties

—even though I have never had the slightest idea what people mean when they talk about the high. Perhaps I don't get high because I have spent most of my life taking drugs that are far more powerful than marihuana.

One evening I smoked marihuana with a friend while playing chess. Tumors in the back of my legs made it difficult for me to sit down for more than five or ten minutes at a stretch. But this time I became so absorbed in the game that I remained sitting for over an hour without any pain. I felt I was in one of those "What's wrong with this picture?" ads. When you are conditioned by pain to be in pain and you suddenly aren't in pain, you immediately start asking why. The only unusual thing I had done was smoke marihuana. I never set out to prove to myself that it helped, but after a while it simply became obvious that even a small amount gave me a quality of pain relief I had never before experienced.

I told my doctor, and he suggested that I use marihuana for six months. If I still felt it was helping me after that, we would discuss it again. For the next six months I smoked marihuana regularly. It not only greatly enhanced the quality of pain relief but drastically decreased my dependence on opioid narcotics and sleeping pills. I became less withdrawn from the world and was able to lead a normal life.

Six months later I reported to my doctor and we discussed the possibility of obtaining marihuana legally. Unfortunately, he died shortly after this conversation, and I was forced to begin searching for a new physician. I wrote to an uncle of mine, a pediatrician who lived in Connecticut. He sent me lots of material on marihuana's medical uses, but said he had no idea whether it could be obtained legally.

I had moved back to Portsmouth, Virginia, where I was brought up, and opened a furniture store. This job kept me on my feet moving furniture all day long. I tore muscles and hemorrhaged almost daily. Occasionally these problems would become very serious. When I received the information from my uncle, I took it to the Portsmouth Police Department and explained my medical

condition to the chief. I told him I could not afford to buy marihuana on the street and asked permission to smoke marihuana
confiscated by the police during raids. The chief said he would
look into it. After speaking with a number of people in town—
Portsmouth is a small city, and my parents are well respected
there—he told me that he could not allow me to use confiscated
marihuana but would tell the men in his department to leave me
alone as long as I did not sell marihuana but bought it only for
medical purposes. There was one other condition—that I never
tell anybody about this informal arrangement. I quickly accepted
the chief's offer and thanked him.

When I walked into my new doctor's office, he made a number of seemingly trivial observations—the little finger on one
hand was unusually large, my arms curved inward, my neck was
short, and so on. He then looked at me and said "pseudopseudohypoparathyroidism." I wondered if he was all there. He pulled
a medical book from a shelf and read me a detailed description
of the disease; it matched perfectly, even the relationship with
multiple congenital cartilaginous exostosis. The doctor suddenly
became very quiet, and I asked him what was wrong. He told me
the bone spurs would continue to grow for the rest of my life,
and any one of them could become malignant at any time. The
resulting cancer would spread quickly and I would die. If cancer
didn't get me, a bone spur might pinch my spinal cord and leave
me a paraplegic, erupt into a major artery and cause me to bleed
to death, or rip into an internal organ and cause permanent, perhaps fatal damage. And the pain would become unbearable.

I asked the doctor if he knew anything about the use of marihuana to control pain and muscle spasticity. He asked me what I
knew. I provided him with the information I'd received from my
uncle. The doctor promised he would review it and said he would
like to follow my case but did not know how he could legally provide me with marihuana. I liked this doctor very much. Not only
was he the first one who actually knew what I had, but he did not
reject outright the notion that marihuana might help. He said that

if I wanted to I could continue smoking and advise him of any difficulties. It was fairly clear, however, that he doubted marihuana's medical value and assumed I was benefiting from a placebo effect.

For the next few years (1976–1979) I continued to smoke marihuana illegally. Although I did not have to fear arrest, the financial drain was serious; I was spending at least three thousand dollars a year on marihuana. My doctor now agreed to help me if I could find out what needed to be done to get legal approval. One condition was that he never be publicly identified. There was too much craziness surrounding the issue, and he was not willing to risk his career by being identified as a "pot doc." He was outraged that as a licensed physician he could prescribe morphine but not marihuana. It was a maddening situation.

He said he didn't have time to complete a lot of forms, construct elaborate research protocols, or attend to all the administrative demands made by the FDA and other federal agencies that control marihuana. But he was willing to sign on the dotted line if I did the leg work, got the forms filled out, and contacted the proper officials. I had no way of knowing just how hard or how slow it would be. It required many hundreds of phone calls and took not weeks or months but years.

The law states that the FDA has thirty days to respond to an Investigational New Drug protocol. Forty-five days after sending my doctor's application we had heard nothing from the FDA, so I called. Officials there politely told me that they had some problems with the IND but could not say what they were; after all, I was only a patient. They would contact my doctor when they were ready. After another long delay, my doctor called, asked the same question, and received the same vague reply. Several months later, after many additional calls from me, the FDA told my doctor what the problems were. All were minor, mostly insignificant. I sensed that the government was hoping to exhaust my doctor and get him to withdraw his request. The FDA clearly had little interest in the IND and even less in my medical welfare.

Approval finally came nearly a year after the initial request, and the first shipment of legal marihuana did not arrive until several months later. We had to perform elaborate tests to determine what benefits I was receiving; for example, once a week I would go to my doctor's office for an electromyogram (EMG), which measures tension and muscle spasticity. After getting a baseline reading, I would leave the office, go to the parking lot, and smoke one or two marihuana cigarettes. Then I would return and take the EMG again.

I have been legally smoking marihuana (2 percent THC) for four and a half years, ten cigarettes a day. I have had a problem with the law only once, at a business meeting in Florida. I was on my feet all day and didn't get a chance to smoke enough marihuana, so my legs were aching by evening. Dinner was to be held in a hotel banquet room. I've never known how to handle this kind of situation, since I don't want to offend people. But I noticed others around me smoking tobacco, and finally decided I had to smoke, too. My wife suggested that I go to the men's room so that I could have some privacy and avoid bothering anyone. While I was there, a busboy came in, noticed the marihuana smell, and asked me if he could take a couple of "hits" from my cigarette. I refused. He became angry and left.

I realized just how angry he was a few minutes later when the men's room was raided by the Orlando Vice Squad. The police rushed in and began asking questions. There was a commotion among my business associates as they led me out of the room. I explained that I was using marihuana supplied by the government, legally, for medical purposes. I was told that it didn't matter since marihuana was illegal under Florida law.

I was placed under arrest and taken to jail. While entering the police station, I tripped on a concrete step, fell, ripped open a blood vessel, and began to hemorrhage. No blood was visible, but my ankle was swelling, and I could not walk. The police officers surrounded me, ordered me to rise, and started pounding their nightsticks into their hands. I began to feel as though I was playing the wrong role in a Grade B movie.

Finally I managed to convince the officers that I could not get up and needed medical help. A nurse was called. She phoned a doctor, who advised her that it didn't sound too bad. My request to be sent to the hospital was rejected. A wheelchair was provided, and I was wheeled in front of a cell. The police confiscated seven pre-rolled NIDA marihuana cigarettes and charged me with possession. Mug shots and fingerprints were taken. I posted bail of $250 and asked for my marihuana cigarettes but was told they were being kept as evidence. I said fine, I had a tin (about 300 cigarettes) in my motel room. By this time the police were obviously beginning to fear that they had made a mistake, since they did not try to obtain a search warrant.

The arrest occurred on a Friday evening. On Monday morning I managed to reach an FDA attorney who said he would "fix things." A short time later the Florida authorities let me know that they would not prosecute and would expunge the record of my arrest. The police returned my bail money but not my marihuana cigarettes.

From my doctor's annual reports to the FDA and my own experience, I know that marihuana has effectively controlled my pain and allowed me to reduce my use of conventional (and far more dangerous) drugs like Sopor, Dilantin, and Dilaudid. The only problem is that NIDA sometimes fails to meet its commitment and provides marihuana of low potency. When that happens, I am forced to smoke so much that my lungs hurt. Otherwise I have never experienced a serious adverse effect.

The value of marihuana in the treatment of pain and other symptoms following brain surgery is described by Karen Ross in the following account:

In 1988 I had surgery for a malignant brain tumor, an oligodendroglioma. The name is as overwhelming as the reality. Two days after the operation I read an article in the *Boston Globe* about the medical uses of marihuana, especially for people undergoing cancer treatments like radiation and chemotherapy. I had been a moderate user of marihuana before my catastrophic illness, and I took serious note of the article, since I was about to have radiation treatments.

After the surgery I was given dexamethasone, an anti-inflammatory drug, for the swelling in my brain, and Zantac [ranitidine] to protect my stomach from the effects of the dexamethasone. Within days after returning home I began to have severe anxiety attacks. Sometimes I thought I would lose my mind. I alternately felt as though my chest was going to burst open or be crushed. My hearing was so acute I could hear the bubbles inside a soda can. My speech was slurred, and I mixed up sounds so that people's words sounded like mumbles unless they were talking directly to me. Often I had to rely on lip reading. For these symptoms the doctor gave me Xanax [alprazolam], a tranquilizer, and Elavil [amitriptyline], an antidepressant. The medications helped somewhat, but I was still not comfortable.

My family obtained some marihuana for me and I began to use it along with the Xanax and Elavil. I would smoke at most two "hits" a couple of times a day. I found that the marihuana relaxed me and focused my attention so that I felt less anxiety and rested more easily. It also relieved the pressure in my head better than dexamethasone. I did not experience a "high." I was already in emotional and physical overdrive, and the marihuana put me at cruising speed, regulated and even. Eventually I was able to reduce my use of Xanax and stop using Elavil entirely.

Six weeks after surgery I started taking radiation treatment and went on taking it five days a week for six weeks. Before and after each treatment I smoked marihuana. It allowed me to sleep during the treatment and took away the tightening and tingling sensation I would otherwise feel in my head afterward.

The dexamethasone caused me to gain sixty-five pounds. I also developed weakness in my muscles, especially in the knees, insomnia, mood swings, personality changes, potassium loss, and facial hair growth. When the dexamethasone was finally withdrawn, six weeks after the radiation treatments ended, I lost most of the weight and regained most of my physical strength. My speech also became clearer (I still have a low tolerance for noise and have to read lips to understand conversations).

All this time I continued to use marihuana. Eventually I returned to part-time work, but shortly afterward marihuana became unavailable. My headache pain, head and eye pressure, facial numbness, anxiety attacks, and slurred speech returned. A brain scan showed no changes in the tumor. When I managed to acquire some marihuana and smoke it, all the symptoms disappeared within a day. A couple of months later marihuana became unavailable again, and my symptoms returned like clockwork. This time I was sure why. Friends were able to find some marihuana and put me back on track again. I started to buy a little here and a little there just to be sure I wouldn't get caught short.

I told my primary-care physician I was taking marihuana for headache pain, pressure, and slurred speech. He told me he couldn't condone it, especially since it was illegal, but he didn't try to stop me. By now I was able to handle my headaches with regular use of Tylenol, Xanax, and marihuana. On the average a single joint would last me three or four days. On some days I didn't smoke at all.

Ten months later I ran out of marihuana again, and the headaches and anxiety returned. I started taking Tylenol with codeine. I was busy packing to move after twelve years of living in my old home, and I thought the stress of moving might have something to do with my problems. I told my oncologist, and he suggested a follow-up brain scan, which showed no change.

Afterward, I met with my neurologist. By this time the pain and pressure in my head were becoming more uncomfortable, and my speech was more slurred. The neurologist concluded that I was having seizures and prescribed Dilantin [diphenylhydantoin, an anticonvulsant], but it didn't help. I only got worse. It caused insomnia, mental confusion, and decreased coordination. I became frustrated and angry. I called the neurologist, and he prescribed dexamethasone again. That didn't help either. He said

I had already had the maximum radiation allowable. This kind of tumor does not respond to chemotherapy, and it was doubtful whether further surgery would be effective. My husband and I left his office feeling as though we had two-hundred-pound bricks on our shoulders. Two days later some friends visited and brought some marihuana. I took two hits. Ten minutes later the pressure behind my eye was gone, I had no more headache, the facial numbness had disappeared, and my speech returned to normal.

Four days after seeing the neurologist, my husband and I visited the oncologist again. He said I might be able to have further radiation treatments, since new technology was available, and surgery could always be used as a last resort. Some of that weight we were carrying on our shoulders was lifted. He noticed that my condition had improved, and I told him about the marihuana. He replied, "I am not going to tell you not to do it, and I am not going to tell you to do it, but if it works, as it obviously does, who am I to say differently?"

We left it at that. I decided to stop taking all the prescribed medications—Dilantin, dexamethasone, and Tylenol with codeine—not only because they weren't working but because I was worried about the side effects. Marihuana didn't have any side effects that I noticed.

The morning after I saw my oncologist, I called the neurologist again. He was pleased that my speech had returned to normal and I sounded more upbeat. I told him it had nothing to do with the drugs he had prescribed, and I was not going to take them any more. He responded as I expected, saying that he didn't approve and that marihuana was illegal. He went on, "If that is what your decision is there is nothing I can do to stop you." My husband and I met him again a couple of weeks later, and I told the story again. He was very critical and demeaning. He told me that I shouldn't drive and that marihuana is damaging to short-term memory. He acted as though I was sitting around getting high all the time. I tried to explain that I smoked only in the morning or evening or when the symptoms were particularly bad and that there was no "high." I think he was reacting this way because I was in control of my care instead of him.

We have decided to find another doctor who isn't so unyielding, narrow-minded, and pessimistic, and, furthermore, is better informed about the new radiation technology. I want to live each day with hope, happiness, and all the zest life can offer. I know my problems are far from over and probably never will be, but I also know I am equipped to manage my life and care, and I refuse to be treated as though I am not. I will continue to recover in my own way with the help of marihuana.

The greatest irony in proscribing the use of cannabis to relieve pain is that the best alternatives are addictive and sometimes debilitating opioids. A woman who described her case to us suffers from melorheostosis, a rare and incurable condition that involves severe joint pain. When she first developed the disorder, her physician prescribed massive doses of Darvocet, a combination of propoxyphene (a synthetic opioid) and Tylenol #3 (codeine and acetaminophen). She needed up to fifteen Darvocets a day to control the pain until she started to smoke marihuana. She has found that "smoking marihuana when the pain first starts will round it off. Otherwise it increases very fast; I begin to feel nauseated and develop cold and hot sweats, simply from the pain." She could usually control the pain with one to two joints a day. "But it is a black-market item, and when we are paying an average of $75 for a quarter of an ounce and you only have an income of $444 a month, you don't buy very much. I feel I should not have to live like a criminal because of the ignorance of politicians. I have to be terrified about whether police will come and search my home. Am I going to lose my home and my children because I have found something that makes me able to cope?"

As a thirty-two-year-old mother of three small children, she found that cannabis did not compromise her functioning the way large doses of opioids did: "Marihuana for some reason relaxes my nervous system and allows me to function mentally on a normal basis. When taking Darvocets and Tylenol I become a different person. I wake up feeling drugged, I go to sleep feeling drugged, I function like a drugged person. I lose little bits and pieces of my family because I am so drugged out that I can't function, even to just sit there and talk to them or read them a story. As a mother I don't have time to lose with my children because of a drug-induced state." This woman echoes the nineteenth-century understanding that cannabis, while it is not as powerful a pain reliever as the opioids, has fewer serious side effects and creates no risk of dependence.

MIGRAINE

Migraine is a severe headache lasting hours to days and accompanied by visual disturbances or nausea and vomiting or both. Usually the attacks are recurrent. They can be brought on in a susceptible person by stress, by certain foods, and by certain types of sensory stimulation (bright light, loud noise, penetrating odors). The onset usually occurs before the age of twenty and rarely after the age of fifty. About 20 percent of the population has experienced migraine attacks; they are three times more common in women than in men.

There are several types of migraine. In common migraine, the pain is usually throbbing and often but not always on one side of the head. It is usually accompanied by nausea and vomiting, and it is exacerbated by any movement or noise. In the comparatively rare classical migraine, the attack begins with visual disturbances (including partial blindness and light flashes in the field of vision) and sometimes dizziness, weakness on one side, ringing in the ears, thirst, drowsiness, or a feeling of impending doom. These neurological symptoms are followed by a severe one-sided headache with sensitivity to light and often nausea and vomiting. Classical migraine may also be complicated by tingling, numbness, weakness, or paralysis in various parts of the body. Another type of headache probably related to migraine is the cluster headache, which is more common in men than in women. In this case the pain is concentrated around one eye; it is constant rather than throbbing, and it usually wakes the sufferer from sleep. It tends to recur nightly for weeks to months and then disappear for months or even years.

Drugs can be used either to cut migraine attacks short or to prevent long-term recurrence. Chemicals derived from ergot, a fungus that grows on rye, are highly effective in stopping an attack at the early stages; ergot derivatives inhibit the effects of serotonin. Once the headache is fully established, opioids (usually codeine or meperidine) can be used to relieve the pain. A relatively new migraine drug is sumatriptan (Imitrex), which also inhibits the effect of serotonin. In general it has fewer side effects than ergotamines, but it causes frightening chest pain in many patients. Furthermore, patients must learn to give themselves subcutaneous injections because sumatriptan is not very effective when taken orally. Other drugs prescribed for prevention of chronic migraine are methysergide (which is related to the ergot derivatives), beta-blockers, calcium channel blockers, chlorpromazine (Thorazine), and the steroid prednisone. Ten to 20 percent of sufferers get no relief from these drugs, and many more get incomplete relief or suffer serious side effects.

As we have noted, cannabis was highly regarded as a treatment for migraine in the nineteenth century, yet the topic is almost untouched in the twentieth-century medical literature. Carol Miller, a classic migraine sufferer, describes her experience as follows:

> I first experienced a migraine in a classroom when I was fourteen. The sparkling, flickering visual effects, which were curious at first, consumed me so that I could not see the blackboard. I asked to be excused, let myself into the nurse's room, and vomited for several hours before my mother came to get me.
>
> After this had happened several times, my mother took me to see our doctor, a close family friend and neighbor whom I saw very often because I had a lot of allergies. He and my mother agreed that the headaches were caused by the recent death of my baby sister, and he gave me nothing for the nausea and pain. Although headaches continued with some regularity,

it wasn't until college that I was given the diagnosis of migraine and received medication. The college infirmary prescribed Ecotrin [coated aspirin], which helped somewhat with the headache but not with the visual effects or the nausea. It also gave me tremendous heartburn.

One time the pain was so severe that they gave me an injection of Demerol [a synthetic opioid], which pretty completely wiped out the pain but left me very lightheaded. At times I took a banana-flavored syrup [probably codeine] which made me very sleepy. I remember that it was difficult to make it through final exams because I was so lightheaded and that my asthma got very bad during this period.

After graduation, while working at Indiana University, I saw a private physician who prescribed Mudrane [a combination including ephedrine and phenobarbital], which he warned was habit-forming. I quit taking them because they seemed to make my blood pressure so low I could hardly work. After moving to San Francisco I was given Darvon [propoxyphene, another opioid], but I took it only briefly because it gave me a rash.

I had been taking aspirin with codeine but found it constipated me terribly. When I became pregnant with my first child, I was very concerned about medication. A friend told me I couldn't take any medication safely and suggested I rely on herbs. I was studying herbal healing and preparing for a natural birth, so this sounded right to me. I tried scullap tea, a light valerian and chamomile tea, and then lavender. The teas were soothing and the slower life pace after quitting work helped; migraines became rare.

Several years later the migraines returned, and my husband said he had read that marihuana was good for headaches. I was amazed. Two hits and a short rest completely warded off the nausea and headache. As soon as I noticed flickering visuals that forewarned me of an approaching migraine, I could take a little cannabis and a short nap and the migraine would not develop at all. I was usually ready to go back to work in a half hour. It gave me a feeling of tremendous power to finally be in such control of my migraines.

In the eighteen years since I began using cannabis to relieve migraines, I have been caught away from home several times without my herb. Once I tried taking Tylenol and found that it helped a little with the pain but not at all with the nausea or the visual effects. Both of my older daughters (now seventeen and twenty-one) also get occasional migraines, which first appeared when they began to menstruate. Both get tremendous relief from cannabis herb. My mother suffers from severe headaches, but she has never used cannabis because it is illegal. She has a horrible time with medications prescribed for her—nausea, constipation, high blood pressure. I often tell her that when marihuana is legal and she uses it for the first time and realizes how she has suffered unnecessarily all these years, she is going to be really furious.

Relief of migraine could be just another analgesic effect of cannabis, but one study suggests that something more is involved. THC has been found to inhibit the release of serotonin from the blood of migraine sufferers during an attack (but not at other times). This result requires confirmation, and its significance remains unclear, but it could be a useful clue to further research.[38]

RHEUMATIC DISEASES

Rheumatic diseases, which are many and diverse, have the common feature of limiting the ability to move freely. Most of them also cause chronic pain and inflammation; marihuana is unquestionably a pain reliever, and it may also be anti-inflammatory.[39] Two common

38. Z. Volfe, A. Dvilansky, and I. Nathan, "Cannabinoids Block Release of Serotonin from Platelets Induced by Plasma from Migraine Patients," *International Journal of Clinical and Pharmacological Research* 5 (1985): 243–246.

39. The anti-inflammatory property may be due to cannabichromene, a nonpsychoactive cannabinoid that has been shown to prevent inflammation in animal experiments. See C. E. Turner and M. A. L. ElSohly, "Biological Activity of Cannabichromene, Its Homologs and Isomers," *Journal of Clinical Pharmacology* 21 (8–9 Suppl.) (August–September 1981): 283S–291S.

forms of rheumatic disease are osteoarthritis and ankylosing spondylitis.

Osteoarthritis

Osteoarthritis is the most common of all joint diseases, affecting 16 million people in the United States alone, including two-thirds of those over sixty-five. It usually develops slowly over many years as the layer of shock-absorbing cartilage that protects the ends of bones breaks down, exposing them and allowing them to grind together. The breakdown of cartilage probably results from poor joint alignment or an accumulation of everyday minor traumatic injuries. The main symptoms are joint stiffness, swelling, and pain, especially in the morning. As the loss of cartilage progresses, irritating the soft tissue around the joint, pain may become constant and interfere with sleep. The disease occurs equally in both men and women; men are affected especially in the hips and back, women in the hands, and both sexes in the knees. The following account is by Kay Lee, an osteoarthritis sufferer who uses marihuana:

> I am fifty-one years old. I have raised five children to productive adulthood pretty much single-handedly and now have four happy grandchildren. I just completed my third year of study toward a BSOP [Business Operations] degree while living alone most of the time. I rather enjoy the challenge. Three years ago I began researching the subject of marihuana as a medicine for a term paper. I chose this topic because, after nearly thirty years of recreational, creative, and therapeutic use, I now relegate most of my cannabis to the medicine cabinet—exactly as my grandmother did before the politicians just said "no."
>
> During my five-year bout with migraines, marihuana replaced Demerol injections many times; for PMS and cramps, it replaced Midol and aspirin; for colds, it replaced expectorants, suppressants, decongestants, antihistamines, and analgesics. When I had to pull myself out of depression after my oldest son drowned, marihuana substituted for Valium and lithium. And now I use it for the chronic pain of arthritis.

Until you or someone you love tries to deal with arthritis, you cannot understand how destructive it is to the quality of life. My mother died at the age of sixty-three, physically much older than her biological age. Doctors couldn't agree on whether she had Alzheimer's or severe depression, but no one misdiagnosed her arthritis. In the last ten years of her life her hands became crippled, deformed, and nearly useless. Hot wax gloves, ace bandages, creams, and pain medications were of no avail. Her tiny, misshapen fingers twisted and curled over each other, some facing the wrong way; her pain was constant and merciless.

For the last couple of years my own hands have begun to take a central place in my life. Doctors tell me an injury triggered a propensity that was already there. I have lost most of the strength in my left hand, and pain in both hands is a loud reminder to limit my movements. The ache involves the knuckles, middle joints, and wrists; cold weather or the slightest injury makes it worse. It is getting hard to lift things and open cans. My fingers become stiff from inaction, from too much action, or from the wrong actions. My sleep is disturbed.

When I smoke what I call "kind medicine," it's never more than three or four minutes before the ache begins to fade. Although it is still there, it seems to have moved into the distance. The physical relief lasts hours longer than the actual high. I try to get a lot done while I am still feeling it.

The ideal dose for me is a half joint every four hours. Since I can't always afford to buy that much, when I have some I limit myself to a half joint twice a day—once in the morning to work and once at night to sleep. When I run out, I simply suffer until I can afford more, and then take on the unpleasant and dangerous task of trying to find cannabis of medicinal quality. I used to worry about people knowing I was high, but no one notices, so I have stopped worrying.

My mother died in despair, robbed of this gentle medicine by politics. She refused to try marihuana because of the misinformation spread by the government and antimarihuana groups. Once my aunt complained to my mother that her son, my cousin, had dropped out of school and was smoking pot. My mother replied, "You know, marihuana makes people stupid." Later I asked her, "Do you think I'm stupid?" she looked at me with astonishment and said, "Of course not." I told her I smoked marihuana. Trembling with fear, she said, "I often thought I would try it if a doctor would make sure nothing went wrong." But no doctor would have helped her, and anyway, my father, with his snapped-shut mind, would have turned us all in. I should have educated her anyway, but I didn't know what I know now. I'm sorry it's too late for her. As for me, I have decided to spread the word for the sake of everyone who needs this medicine or cares about someone who could benefit from it.

Ankylosing Spondylitis

Ankylosing spondylitis usually strikes young adults, affecting about 300,000 people in the United States, three-fourths of whom are men. It is a chronic inflammatory disease that attacks joint cartilage and entheses, the points where ligaments and tendons are inserted into bones. Eventually bone replaces soft tissue and joints are fused, especially in the spine and the pelvis. Sometimes ossification involves the entire spine and pulls it out of alignment. In other cases cervical (neck) vertebrae are fused and turning the head becomes difficult. Pain is constant; it is worse in the morning, at night, and after periods of inactivity. The following account was written by a sixty-year-old man who suffers from ankylosing spondylitis:

One day in the early 1950s I started out for school in my old 1932 Plymouth, but the battery was dead. My father and I pushed the car to get it started; I hurt my back in the process and have had problems ever since. In 1955, while I was in the Navy, the pain became so bad that my stride was limited to ten inches and I could not even find a comfortable position to sleep. After intensive examination at a naval hospital, I was told there was nothing wrong with my back and I was a goldbrick. I informed them in no uncertain terms that I had signed on for four years and intended to complete my contract. They released me back to the base. A few weeks later the pain became bearable, and I completed my tour of duty.

In 1963 or 1964 I was diagnosed with rheumatoid arthritis and treated accordingly with medication and physical therapy. In 1973, while living in California, I was introduced to marihuana by a woman I had invited on a date. I smoked a little and found that as the evening wore on, the pain with which I constantly lived became mute.

At that time a lid [ounce] of marihuana cost five dollars. I'll never forget when it rose to ten dollars. I wasn't sure it was worth it, so I quit. The pain returned with an intensity I had forgotten, so I soon began paying the required price.

In 1981 my new wife and I moved from California to the southern Rocky Mountain region where I was brought up. I ran out of marihuana, and it took a while to find a connection so that I could once more live with limited pain.

By now my spine had solidified from the base of my neck to the top of my tail bone; it had the elasticity of a broom handle. One medical practitioner took an X-ray and said, "I'd never have believed it had I not seen it." I received a new diagnosis: ankylosing spondylitis. Now that my spine has solidified, my pain is not quite so severe, but it is constant. If kidney stones are ten on a pain scale, my pain varies from three to seven, depending on the weather and the barometric pressure. Tolectin [tolmetin, a nonsteroidal anti-inflammatory drug] is helpful, but marihuana still provides the best relief.

I have earned a B.A., two M.A.s, and a Ph.D., and I have received an honorary LL.D. When last measured my I.Q. registered 145. I know when I have found something that will improve my life.

Patients with arthritic disorders are usually treated with either acetaminophen (Tylenol) or one of the nonsteroidal anti-inflammatory drugs, such as ibuprofen, naproxen, or aspirin. We have already discussed the toxic side effects of these drugs. When cannabis becomes legally available, it will be less expensive and risky than either acetaminophen or NSAIDs.

Atopic dermatitis is an inflammatory skin disorder that is probably an allergic reaction of unknown origin. The symptoms are pruritus (severe itching) and patches of inflamed skin, especially on the hands, face, neck, legs, and genitals. It is usually treated with corticosteroids and ointments applied to the skin. Steroids are only partially effective and in any case can be used only occasionally during crises, since long-term use has serious side effects. Antihistamines help to control the itching, but they too have limited value. In serious cases, the scratching causes infections that must be treated with antibiotics. Don Spear, a sixty-year-old man from Flint, Michigan, tells the following story:

> I am afflicted with a debilitating, potentially life-threatening skin condition called atopic neurodermatitis. In 1954, as an eighteen-year-old, while stationed at an Army base in Texas, I noticed that the skin around my eyes was itchy and scaling. At first I thought it was the arid Texas climate, but the condition became worse and spread to other parts of my body. The skin in affected areas became highly irritated, turned dark red, and began to split open. A year later, when the Army transferred me to West Germany, much of my body was covered with patches of blistered, bright red skin that would split open, scab, and split open again. These areas became infected from constant scratching.
>
> Doctors in Army hospitals in Germany diagnosed my condition as atopic neurodermatitis. I used all the available medications, ointments, and preparations, but nothing helped. My hands and arms were shredded from split, scabbing skin and constant scratching. Gangrene set in, and the doctors considered

amputating both my arms at the elbow. In a last effort to prevent amputation, my forearms were completely bandaged so that I could not scratch them; I was also given massive doses of antibiotics and the new "wonder drug," cortisone. For the itching, which nearly drove me out of my mind, the doctors prescribed tranquilizers and sedatives. My arms were saved, but I could not tolerate any more cortisone. Despite the Army's best efforts, my skin condition could not be controlled. In January 1956, I was discharged with a 50 percent service-connected disability.

In the next ten years I tried nearly every available prescription and over-the-counter drug: heavy doses of Librium, Valium, and other addictive tranquilizers, cortisone creams and ointments, coal tar baths and preparations. None provided long-term relief. I was hospitalized several times because of infections that resulted from uncontrollable itching and split skin.

Because my skin condition was disfiguring, it was difficult to find work. Employers would not hire me, and other workers did not want to work with me. I finally took a job with the Fisher Body Company, but I repeatedly needed prolonged sick leave. After ten years the company computed that I had taken six years of sick leave and retired me. Looking for work to support my wife and four children, I again discovered that many people simply would not hire me. The skin disease persisted. I would often wake up at night and find that blood had oozed from my scalp onto the pillow. The itching was so severe and intense that I used sandpaper on my skin to get relief. My marriage broke up, and I became very withdrawn and frightened.

In the spring of 1973, a friend who had served in Vietnam told me that he had smoked marihuana there and found it enjoyable. I was reluctant, not only because it was illegal but also because I did not like to use drugs of any kind. I had long since given up alcohol and tobacco, and my experience with prescription drugs made me even more cautious. I come from a strict, moral background in which drug use is regarded as not right.

Finally, one weekend at a drag race, I took a few puffs from

my friend's marihuana cigarette. I may also have taken a couple
of puffs from another cigarette the next day. I noticed nothing
unusual after smoking, no mental effects. On Tuesday or Wednes-
day of the following week I realized that a particularly bad area
of skin looked much less red and inflamed. It occurred to me
that the itching had not been bothering me for several days. I
wondered whether marihuana had anything to do with the unexpected improvement but did not give the idea much credit.

The next weekend my friend and I went to another drag race,
and he offered me marihuana again. By this time the itching had
returned, but it stopped suddenly with the first puff. I was astonished. After years of my using every drug and skin product
available without gaining relief, the itching stopped with one puff
of a marihuana cigarette. For the next three years I continued
to smoke marihuana only on weekends, and never more than a
few puffs at a time. My skin condition improved dramatically.
Because I was no longer scratching, the split skin healed. Then
the red patches began to fade and were replaced by normal skin.
Soon I was no longer disfigured. I got a regular job and became
a solid worker. I no longer had to take sick leave.

In early 1977 my older brothers discovered that I was smoking
marihuana and told our parents. Although I was over forty, I
cared very deeply for their feelings. I explained the situation to
them, but I could see they were not convinced. They feared that
I had become addicted. I told them I would stop smoking marihuana for three months and see what happened. I had never
experienced any adverse mental or physical effects, and I had no
difficulty quitting. I developed no craving and had no "shakes"
or "sweats." But within three days my entire body was itching.
The skin between my toes and fingers became irritated and inflamed. The inflammation quickly spread up my hands and feet
to my arms and legs, then to my scalp, head, and chest. Within
weeks my skin was splitting, I was scratching constantly, and
dark red welts appeared over much of my body. I was becoming
disfigured again, and there was blood on the sheets at night. My

parents and brother became alarmed and pleaded with me to start smoking marihuana again. I was reluctant because I did not like to be called an addict. Finally I realized that my family did not care whether marihuana was illegal. They only cared about its effect on my skin.

I began smoking on weekends again. This time it took nearly a year before my skin was back to normal. I continued to smoke marihuana for the next decade, until February 1987, and my skin condition remained under control. I maintained a good employment record and never smoked while working. In February 1987, I learned that my company intended to conduct random urinalysis tests on its employees. I requested help from my union representatives and meanwhile asked doctors at the Veterans' Administration to help me obtain marihuana legally. They referred me to the VA Drug Rehabilitation Unit, where I was told that I did not have a drug problem. In effect, the doctors there decided that I was simply using the drug therapeutically. They encouraged me to continue smoking marihuana. But the threat of urine testing and the possible loss of my job deeply upset me. Confused, not knowing what to do, I stopped smoking. My skin condition almost immediately erupted.

After a few weeks it was serious and rapidly growing worse. My parents, my brother, good friends, and even my union representative encouraged me to start smoking marihuana again. The alternative was to obey the law and live with a deforming skin condition that might, through infection, kill me. I took sick leave and started to grow my own marihuana.

In December 1989 a neighbor told the police. I was arrested and convicted. The punishment was a large fine, house arrest for four months, and two years of probation. The judge said that all charges would be dropped if I obtained a legal prescription. But I have had to stop smoking because of the urine tests at work. Since I stopped again (December 1989), the itching has been almost constant, and my skin repeatedly splits open and leaks fluid on my feet, hands, scalp, legs, chest, and even penis.

Marihuana is the only drug that prevents both the skin lesions and the horrible itching. If marihuana were legal, I could control this hell of a disease. Marihuana might also help thousands of people with similar skin problems, but there is no research because it is a prohibited drug and doctors do not like political controversy.

PREMENSTRUAL SYNDROME, MENSTRUAL CRAMPS, AND LABOR PAINS

The symptoms of premenstrual syndrome (PMS), which occurs in some women during the week before menstruation, include anxiety, sadness, irritability, fatigue, moodiness, difficulty in concentrating, and various physical discomforts.

Cannabis was commonly used in the nineteenth century for the treatment of symptoms associated with the menstrual cycle. J. R. Reynolds, Queen Victoria's physician, prescribed it to her for premenstrual symptoms and menstrual cramps. In 1890 he wrote in *The Lancet*, England's premier medical journal: "When pure and administered carefully it [cannabis] is one of the most valuable medicines we possess."[40]

Although there is no twentieth-century medical literature on the topic, many women with premenstrual syndrome say that they find cannabis useful. Judy Fix is a thirty-five-year-old administrative assistant to a Wall Street broker:

I have used marihuana for many years to alleviate the symptoms of premenstrual syndrome—bloating, headaches, mood swings, and anxiety. I also use it to relieve cramping and fatigue during the menstrual cycle itself. I have tried conventional medicines such as aspirin, acetaminophen, and ibuprofen. Only ibuprofen has any effect; it eliminates cramping, but only in a triple dose that causes increased bloating, drowsiness, and constipa-

40. J. R. Reynolds, "Therapeutic Uses and Toxic Effects of *Cannabis Indica*," *Lancet* (March 22, 1890): 637–638.

tion. When I start to experience the confusion, anger, and hypersensitivity that signal the onset of a premenstrual mood swing, smoking a joint is the one remedy that works immediately to soothe my nerves. It is as if my whole system has been slowed to put everything in order. My thought processes are less jumbled; I react less impulsively and become more rational. If I smoke half a joint at night, I sleep better. My husband of six years has attested to these effects many times.

For the last five years I have worked in a fast-paced and tense environment that requires me to keep a clear head and make important decisions. On a normal day smoking pot might be detrimental to my performance, but when I'm premenstrual it becomes necessary if I am to function at my usual capacity. I'll go outside and take a few hits off a joint, and by the time I return I feel much more in control. I'm able to organize my work and think each task through. I usually smoke at two-hour intervals. My employer and some of my co-workers are aware of the situation, and they support me fully, even though they do not smoke marihuana themselves. I recently gave a woman at my workplace a joint during her menstrual period, and she came in the next morning raving about how it eased her cramps and decreased her anxiety.

Recently my husband was charged with possession of marihuana. He had just bought some at a local grocery, and we were stopped by undercover cops as we drove away. The police drew their guns, put us up against a wall, and threatened my husband with a beating. After speaking with us and seeing that we were reasonable people, they told us they had to arrest him to help close down the store. We were told that he would be held for a few hours and then issued a summons, which they said would probably be thrown out of court.

The whole experience made me angry. Both we and the officers were put in a compromising position. If pot were legal, the police could concentrate on more serious issues. Meanwhile, I still have to worry about losing my job if the wrong person sees me smoking. I am not a menace to society but a productive person seeking relief from a very real medical problem. The benefits of marihuana greatly outweigh the risks; I have found nothing else as effective and nonirritating. I hope the medical community will grow more assertive in supporting the legalization of medical marihuana.

Selective serotonin reuptake inhibitors (SSRIs) such as fluoxetine (Prozac) have been shown to be an effective treatment for severe PMS, but they often have side effects, including loss of sexual desire, that may limit their use, and they may not work for all women with the disorder. Further clinical investigation of cannabis is warranted.

Although, as we point out elsewhere, pregnant and nursing women should generally avoid drugs, there are cases in which the need is so great and the benefits so far outweigh the risks that an exception is appropriate.

As the following account indicates, marihuana can be used to relieve not only menstrual cramps but also nausea during pregnancy and labor pains:

I am a thirty-seven-year-old housewife. I run a small business, volunteer in my daughters' school, and chaperone class trips. I appear to be "straight," and many of my neighbors and acquaintances have no idea I smoke marihuana. I have had painful menstrual cramps for many years, and in 1976 a laparoscopy revealed ovarian cysts and endometriosis. I was told that the endometriosis would return after an operation, so I decided not to have one. I took hormone shots for several months but stopped because I was afraid of cancer. Prescription painkillers made me feel too drugged to function efficiently as a mother. At that time I used pot as a recreational drug, smoking it socially with friends, and I accidentally found out that it also relieved my menstrual cramps. Now most of my friends don't even know I smoke, but I light up as soon as my menstrual period starts.

I had my first baby in 1972, when I was only seventeen. The doctors gave me a shot to put me to sleep, and when I woke up

I had a very lethargic baby. We spent three days in the hospital. In 1979, when I had my second baby, I went to natural childbirth classes and later smoked pot on the way to the hospital. It greatly relaxed me and thus relieved some of the pain, but the effect lasted only about an hour and a half. I was in the hospital for only twenty hours this time, and I was amazed at how much more alert and hungry the second baby was compared to my poor drugged first baby.

In 1991 I became pregnant again. In my seventh month, I became nauseous, had heartburn, and began to vomit two to four times a day—so much that I wasn't gaining weight. The doctor decided the cause was pressure from the baby on the valve at the top of my stomach. I began smoking pot before meals, and after that I vomited only twice a week. The baby weighed nine pounds at birth. I wonder how small she would have been if I hadn't used my favorite antinausea drug.

This time when I had the baby I stayed home and smoked pot for the first seven hours of labor. I delivered less than three hours after arriving at the hospital and the pain was no problem until the pot wore off, just before I delivered. This time I was not surprised that the baby was alert and hungry. We went home six hours after birth; I spent less than nine hours at the hospital, and wasn't even billed for a whole day.

DEPRESSION AND OTHER MOOD DISORDERS

For most people, depression is a passing mood; for some, it is a debilitating chronic illness with severe physical as well as emotional symptoms. When it is deep and persistent enough to interfere with work, friendships, family life, or even physical health, depression is regarded as a psychiatric disorder—one of the most common and one of the most serious.

An episode of severe, or major, depression may last several weeks to several years. One set of symptoms is inconsolable misery accompanied by despair and guilt. Victims feel worthless and inadequate;

they have no hope for the future and ruminate about death and suicide. They may think that they have lost all their money or are being punished for grave sins or are dying of incurable diseases. Some depressed persons do not admit sadness or guilt; instead, they withdraw from human contacts, lose all interest in life, and become incapable of feeling pleasure. Time passes slowly for them, and the world seems dreary and meaningless. Normal emotional responses, even ordinary despondency or grief, become impossible. They are fretful and irritable. They cannot concentrate or make even minor decisions. They turn the same few ideas over and over in their minds. Some depressed patients are listless and lethargic, with slow movements, toneless speech, and an expressionless face—in extreme cases, muteness and immobility resembling catatonic stupor. Others pace, weep, moan, and wring their hands in anxious agitation.

Depression is not simply a disorder of mood. Depressed people lack energy in every sense, physical as well as emotional and intellectual. The dominant symptoms may be loss of appetite and insomnia (or, sometimes, oversleeping and a ravenous appetite), backaches, headaches, upset stomachs, constipation, and above all chronic fatigue. People who claim to be "tired all the time" may be depressed even if they acknowledge no sadness or despair. Manic persons, on the other hand, are sleepless and tireless—until they become exhausted and break down.

The standard treatments for depression are the many antidepressant drugs introduced in the past forty years. For a long time the most popular group of antidepressants was the tricyclics, including imipramine (Tofranil), amitriptyline (Elavil), desipramine (Norpramin), and several other drugs. Their most common side effects are dry mouth and blurred vision. Others are weight gain, constipation, difficulty in urinating, and orthostatic or postural hypotension (dizziness caused by a reduced blood flow to the brain on sitting up or standing up). They can be risky for patients with cardiovascular disease because they increase the heart rate and may disturb cardiac rhythm.

Another group of antidepressants is the monoamine oxidase (MAO) inhibitors: isocarboxazid (Marplan), tranylcypromine (Parnate), and phenelzine (Nardil). They may cause dizziness, insomnia, and impotence, and when used in combination with such foods as red wine, pickles, and certain cheeses which contain the substance tyramine can produce dangerously high blood pressure. Because of these potentially serious side effects, they are rarely the first choice in treating depression, but they may be helpful for patients who do not improve on other drugs.

An increasingly popular new group of antidepressants with fewer and less serious side effects is the selective serotonin reuptake inhibitors (SSRIs). The most popular of these drugs are fluoxetine (Prozac), sertraline (Zoloft), and paroxetine (Paxil). Their side effects include nausea, weight loss, agitation (or, in some cases, drowsiness), and loss of sexual interest or capacity.

In bipolar or manic-depressive disorder, the inconsolable misery of major depression alternates with mania or uncontrolled elation. In the manic phase people with bipolar disorder are cheerful, gregarious, talkative, energetic, and hyperactive. Their spending is often extravagant and their behavior reckless. They may imagine that they have extraordinary talents and are or soon will be rich and powerful. This restless cheerfulness and expansiveness can suddenly turn into incoherent agitation, irritability, rage, paranoia, or grandiose delusions.

Antidepressants alone are not a good treatment for bipolar disorder and may even make it worse. Lithium carbonate, introduced into medicine at about the same time as tricyclics, has revolutionized the treatment of bipolar disorder. It prevents mania and to a lesser extent bipolar depression. Although lithium takes several weeks to start working, its success rate is about 70 percent, and 20 percent of patients are completely freed of their symptoms. Patients generally require long-term maintenance treatment, and because lithium can be toxic it must be used carefully. Chronic use may endanger the heart, kidneys, and thyroid gland. Usually the dose is gradually increased until the drug begins to work and then periodically readjusted according to the patient's age, medical condition, and psychiatric symptoms. The amount of lithium in the blood must be checked regularly because it is ineffective if too low and risky if too high. Some side effects are weight gain, hand tremors, drowsiness, and excessive thirst or urination. Patients often cannot tolerate lithium either because of the side effects or because it takes some of the joy from their lives along with the manic episodes. It has been described as a "loose-fitting emotional straitjacket." Only 20 percent of patients with bipolar disorder take lithium alone. Other drugs used in the treatment of bipolar disorder are the anticonvulsants carbamazepine (Tegretol) and valproic acid (Depakote), which may be used either alone or in combination with lithium.

Cannabis first appeared in the Western medical literature as a suggested treatment for depression in the middle of the nineteenth century. In 1845, Jacques-Joseph Moreau de Tours proposed its use in melancholia (especially with obsessive rumination) and chronic mental illness in general.[41] Over the next hundred years medical papers supported and disputed the utility of cannabis in the treatment of depression. In 1947 G. T. Stockings, an English physician, administered a synthetic THC to fifty depressed patients, and thirty-six showed definite improvement. Obsessive ruminations were significantly reduced in six out of seven patients.[42] In 1948, D. A. Pond failed to replicate these results.[43] In 1950 C. S. Parker and F. W. Wrigley conducted a double-blind study involving fifty-seven patients suffering from severe melancholia or milder depression and found no difference between the synthetic THC and a placebo, but they used a smaller dose than Stockings, 10–20 mg as opposed to 15–90 mg.[44]

The most recent study on cannabis and depression was undertaken in 1973. Eight hospitalized patients were given either THC or a placebo for up to a week. The THC did not relieve their depression, and

41. J.-J. Moreau de Tours, "Lypemanie avec stupeur; tendance à la démence. —traitement par l'extrait (principe resineux) de cannabis indica—Guérison," *Lancette Gazette Hôpital* 30 (1857): 391.

42. G. T. Stockings, "A New Euphoriant for Depressive Mental States," *British Medical Journal* 1 (1947): 918–922.

43. D. A. Pond, "Psychological Effects in Depressive Patients of the Marihuana Homologue Synhexyl," *Journal of Neurology, Neurosurgery and Psychiatry* 11 (1948): 279.

44. C. S. Parker and F. W. Wrigley, "Synthetic Cannabis Preparations in Psychiatry: I. Synhexyl," *Journal of Mental Science* 96 (1950): 276–279.

in four of the patients it produced discomfort and anxiety so serious it had to be withdrawn. The authors questioned whether "different effects might be observed in other settings or in patients with less severe depressive symptoms." They also noted that "the administration of THC under double-blind conditions in this trial precluded the establishment of any positive expectations in the patient. The fact that the patients could not have prepared themselves for the experience of an altered state of consciousness may also have contributed to the predominantly negative effects of the drug in these depressed patients. Finally, the relatively brief duration of the trial (one week) must be kept in mind since standard antidepressants require two to three weeks to produce clinical improvement."[45]

Today, among the minority of depressed patients who do not respond to any of the standard antidepressants or who find the side effects unbearable, some have discovered that cannabis is more useful than any legal drug. We first learned about the following patient's use of cannabis from her psychiatrist. She called us because she was puzzled to find that marihuana was more useful than the drugs she had prescribed, and she wanted to be reassured of its safety. The patient gives her account below:

> I am a thirty-nine-year-old health professional who suffers from chronic depression. I have been able to graduate from college, receive a postgraduate degree with highest honors, and establish a successful professional career, but it has been a constant struggle. No matter how much I accomplished, how much praise I received, none of it registered. I could only ruminate about my shortcomings, and I seemed to have no control over my unrealistic negative thoughts.
>
> My first major episode of depression occurred in 1969, when I went away to college. I withdrew halfway through my freshman year and began semi-weekly therapy sessions with a psychiatrist. With her help and the use of a tricyclic antidepressant, I was able

45. J. Kotin, R. M. Post, and F. K. Goodwin, "Delta-9-tetrahydrocannabinol in Depressed Patients," *Archives of General Psychiatry* 28 (1973): 345–348.

to return to a college closer to home the following September. I continued to see her once a week until I left the East in August 1976. While at school in the Midwest, I saw a psychiatrist renowned for his expertise in the pharmacological treatment of depression. Since I returned to the East in 1981, I have been in therapy once again with my original psychiatrist, either once a week or every two weeks.

Under the guidance of these therapists I have tried more than a dozen different drugs, including several types of tricyclic anti-depressants, Prozac, lithium, Ritalin [methylphenidate, a stimulant related to amphetamine], synthetic thyroid hormone, and probably others I have forgotten. The only ones that have affected my moods significantly are Elavil at high doses and combinations of Dexedrine [dextroamphetamine] and a barbiturate. Elavil works only during an incapacitating episode of depression, and its side effects, especially constipation, are distressing. Since the use of Dexedrine and barbiturates as antidepressants is considered unorthodox, my therapist and I have been uneasy about it, but it was the only medication that worked. Several prominent psychiatrists have verified this and recommended that I use whatever helps. But now I am becoming tolerant to both of these drugs (I have been careful not to increase the dose, because I know the dangers).

In the spring of 1990 I smoked marihuana for the first time since 1973. To my amazement, a quarter of a joint changed my self-perception to match the person others saw. It was like night and day. I had experienced a similar change only a few times before, when Elavil kicked in and lifted me out of the depths. But with Elavil it took four days of rapidly increasing doses; with marihuana it took less than five minutes, every time. Since then I have been using marihuana to think clearly, to concentrate, and simply to enjoy the beauty of the world in a way I couldn't for years.

I try to carry the same positive feelings with me while I am not directly under the influence of marihuana. I now use marihuana as an antidepressant once or at most twice a day. No one realizes I am smoking it because I don't act stoned. I have been cutting back on my other medications and often forget to take them. After smoking some cannabis in the morning, I no longer dread the responsibility of going to work but actually look forward to it. I have always awakened in the morning more exhausted than when I went to sleep. Even during weekends and vacations, I have found it difficult to get dressed and get moving. Immediately after I smoke marihuana, all that changes. I feel energetic and loquacious; I want to socialize, exercise, or do whatever needs to be done. I feel a passion for life. I even see myself differently in the mirror and realize that I am not the homely beast I usually see. While using marihuana I realized that I was not spending time with the person I wanted to be with, so I ended an unsatisfying relationship of two and a half years. I am now with someone I love dearly. Without marihuana I have an orgasm only through masturbation or after heroic efforts during intercourse. Cannabis transforms me into a fully developed sexual human being. I can easily shut out inappropriate thoughts and enjoy what I am feeling. I can have orgasms by stimulation practically anywhere on my body, even just through kissing—amazing!

It is unfair and cruel that the antidepressant that helps me most (and is probably, in its pure form, least toxic) is unavailable for legal prescription. I have to break the law to obtain it and pay exorbitant prices for a drug whose cost of production is minimal.

Another patient who suffers from episodic depression writes as follows:

I am a forty-seven-year-old white male, a partner in a multi-million dollar company. . . . As soon as I started school my emotional problems became apparent, and an endless trek to various health professionals began. My school phobia made me sneak away from school, sometimes by climbing out windows. I spent much time being interviewed by "special ed" teachers and social workers. From early on I was examined by a continuous flow of physicians. My earliest recollection is of the one who prescribed special arches for my shoes (to relieve headaches) and a syrup at night to make me sleep.

The headaches persisted; the depressions became paralyzing episodes that occurred several times a year and lasted days to weeks. Because of them I missed much of grade school and junior high.

In my sophomore year of high school things got worse. I was given a prescription for Miltown [meprobamate, an anti-anxiety drug]. I took it in varying dosages for several months. It caused me to become drowsy and dizzy; my speech slurred, and I developed chronic diarrhea. My poor performance in school worsened. I started to lose my coordination. My depressions continued, perhaps made worse. I was glad to stop using it.

My experience with Miltown was so unpleasant that I refused to take any other "mental" drugs for the next two years. I did see a therapist on a weekly basis. His diagnosis was "episodes of acute depression."

During this period I managed to just barely complete high school and got accepted at a small local college. During my second semester I attempted suicide. I was told by a doctor that I had an "obsessive-compulsive personality." It was suggested that I take Librium. I started taking this drug and found myself in a continuing state of depression, confusion, and lethargy. I had to leave school. When my speech started slurring, I abandoned the Librium.

I got a job driving a truck, and started seeing a new doctor, a psychiatrist. After nine months I reapplied to college and was accepted. The doctor convinced me to try another drug, Tofranil, that he said was very effective in treating depression. I started using it and soon found I was losing all power of concentration. I became restless, full of anxiety. It became almost impossible to urinate. I developed a lump the size of a marble in my left nipple. The doctor ascribed these symptoms to the Tofranil. I stopped using it and again left school. My depression was still there, and

I was desperate for some relief. I also started getting pains in my stomach. A GI series revealed a duodenal ulcer. I constantly chewed antacids and took tablets called Zantac [ranitidine, an ulcer treatment].

Life was becoming more difficult, and the doctor suggested another medicine, Vivactil [protriptyline, a tricyclic antidepressant]. Again, the side effects were disastrous. I became more agitated than before, had great trouble urinating, and a chronic skin disease I have (atopic dermatitis) started to itch with a fury. I developed a peculiar taste in my mouth that would not leave and had a continual feeling of nausea. Shortly after discontinuing Vivactil I was in the psychiatric ward of a New York hospital, suffering from "atypical depression."

In the hospital I was put on lithium. After two days my hands started to shake. This tremor became so intense that after one week I was unable to write or hold a glass without spilling the contents. I had diarrhea and nausea; my vision started to blur.

I ceased using the lithium and left the hospital after a stay of two weeks. When I saw my therapist again he made an unusual statement: "I'm not suggesting this," he said, "if I did I could lose my license, but have you ever tried marihuana?" I had smoked something alleged to be marihuana once in high school and had been unaffected. I thought it might be worth another try. I called a friend I suspected would know where or how to obtain some, and the next day she brought me two joints. I later learned that her husband (who is a dentist) used marihuana to ease the pain of chronic depression.

Remembering my previous experience, I had low expectations. Alone in my room I lit the first joint. Soon I found myself lost in reverie. Previously, when I was depressed, the sadness became the focal point of my existence. Now my mind was being distracted by neutral and even funny or pleasant thoughts. The constant pain of the depression was reduced to an occasional nagging ache. I slept well and awoke feeling refreshed, not "doped up" and lethargic. It soon became apparent that when I was in the throes of a depressive episode, a marihuana cigarette was a greater source of relief than anything I had ever tried before—not a cure, but something that diluted the pain. The marihuana permitted me to function better than any licit drug. I didn't become drowsy, develop tremors, or have any of the side effects associated with the drugs I had previously taken. I gained an appetite I never had and put needed weight on an emaciated frame. I found myself having ideas that would not ordinarily have come to me, some practical, some not. I was able to pierce the black cloud that surrounded me and climb out far enough to meet my responsibilities. The use of marihuana makes it impossible for depressive thoughts to become the total focus of my life.

The fact that marihuana is illegal made me search for a licit medicine that was at least as effective. The next one I was given was Norpramin. This chemical offered no relief and came with an assortment of side effects that aggravated my prostate, gave me diarrhea, left a terrible, lingering taste in my mouth, and colored my tongue black. For about a year I was given Adapin [doxepin, another tricyclic] with only minor side effects, but it did little or nothing to change my condition. I was also given Buspar [buspirone, an anti-anxiety drug], which seems to have no effect at all. Perhaps the very worst of them all was Prozac, which actually made me more anxious, nauseous, dizzy to the point of fainting, and unable to achieve orgasm. I have also had Desyrel [trazodone], which causes only minor side effects, but again seems to do little good.

As of this writing, I have smoked marihuana for more than two decades. In addition to dampening the pain of depression, I have found that it reduces nausea and burning in the stomach due to the production of acid. It allows me to sleep peacefully. It stimulates my imagination when working on creative projects. It enhances simple joys, such as eating M&Ms or walking in the woods. Since its use jeopardizes my freedom, I would prefer a legal substitute. So far I have found none.

I use no other illicit substances. I do not use tobacco. My alcohol intake is no more than an occasional drink on a Saturday night out. I usually have one cup of tea a day and two glasses of Coca-Cola. I take several aspirins a week.

Ron Leifer, M.D., is a psychiatrist who practices in Ithaca, New York. He reports on two of his patients who found cannabis useful for the treatment of depression:

> In more than thirty years of practicing psychiatry in a small university town, I have encountered many patients who use marihuana, and in most cases this use is unrelated to the problem for which they seek therapy. But a few of my patients have used marihuana for the relief of chronic depression, as the following examples indicate.
>
> Mr. T was a forty-four-year-old history teacher at a local college who came in looking unhappy and complaining about all aspects of his life — his work, his marriage, his house, his finances. He said he saw no hope of improving his situation. He was angry, cynical, and critical of others. He stated half in jest that he often thought of committing homicide or suicide. He asked for medication to relieve his depression.
>
> Mr. T's father was a Polish Jew who escaped before World War II, while his own father died at Auschwitz. He worked as an upholsterer in Florida. The patient was terrified of his stern father but also greatly loved him. In 1958, when the patient was eight years old, his father became depressed and was given electroshock therapy. He died of a heart attack five years later, when the patient was fourteen, and Mr. T traces his own depression to that time.
>
> He first consulted a psychiatrist in 1970 and since then has been given Desyrel [trazodone], Elavil [amitriptyline], Prozac [fluoxetine], Wellbutrin [bupropion], lithium, and three or four other antidepressants whose names he cannot remember. None of them brought relief. He first tried marihuana in 1986, when he was in Amsterdam with his wife and her dance troupe. It gave him immediate relief, but he was reluctant to continue using it because it irritated his lungs.

The day after his initial consultation, Mr. T called for an emergency appointment and begged for anxiety medication. I prescribed Valium [diazepam]. At the next meeting a week later he said he did not like Valium and asked for an antidepressant. I now prescribed Prozac [fluoxetine] along with Xanax [alprazolam] for anxiety. He said the Prozac made him jumpy and within a month had stopped taking it. He now asked for Marinol, saying he did not want to smoke marihuana because he feared the legal consequences and because it aggravated his bronchial problems.

I arranged a consultation with Dr. Grinspoon, who prescribed Marinol, 5 mg twice a day. Three days later the patient called to say he was feeling much better. He was more energetic and thinking more clearly. A month later he reported that he felt great; his depression was gone, his negative thoughts had disappeared, and he was no longer cranky and angry. He loved his work, he was getting along with his wife, and he was sleeping well. Since he was no longer anxious, he had stopped taking Xanax. Three months after the initial consultation he described Marinol (which he was now taking three times a day) as a "miracle drug."

After six months his insurance ran out and he was unable to afford Marinol. He turned to street marihuana, although he was unhappy about this because of the expense and the bronchial irritation. Then he was granted Medicaid and asked me to prescribe Marinol again, but I was reluctant because I could not get prior approval and feared the reaction of the state government. Mr. T is still successfully using street marihuana to treat his depression.

Mr. F, a sixty-five-year-old retired college professor, was referred by a psychopharmacologist from New York City. Dr. Grinspoon had recommended Marinol, and the patient was looking for a physician closer to his home who would prescribe it for him.

Mr. F said that he had been depressed for the past twenty years. He had been in psychotherapy all that time with a local psychiatrist who says that he suffers from "characterological depression." He had been unsuccessfully treated with a variety of antidepressants, including Prozac, Tofranil [imipramine], and desipramine. He had been in psychiatric hospitals several times, and nine months before seeing me he had received ECT [electroconvulsive treatment], which was also ineffective.

When he first tried marihuana, in 1975, it had no effect. But later it was given to him by fellow patients on the psychiatric ward of a local hospital, producing "the first authentic depression-free moment of my life." He did not want to use marihuana habitually because it was difficult to obtain and legally risky, and he was worried about the effect on his heart and lungs. He says the Marinol prescribed by Dr. Grinspoon gave him instant relief from his depression. He calls it "a miracle drug."

He had an angioplasty in July of this year [1993] and since that time has been following a strict low-fat diet with yogic exercises. He has chronic atrial fibrillation, for which he has refused all prescribed medication.

After consulting with Dr. Grinspoon, I prescribed 5 mg of Marinol three times a day. The patient says he is no longer depressed and suffers from no confusion, memory loss, or other negative side effects.

Thirty to forty percent of patients with bipolar disorder are not consistently helped by conventional treatment. For some of them cannabis may be useful in ameliorating the symptoms, reducing the side effects of lithium, or both. The following account is written by a forty-six-year-old woman with apparent bipolar disorder:

I was born on Friday, October 13, 1950, a few months before my father had his first serious bout with manic depression. My mother said he was taking valuable art objects they owned and throwing them down the trash chute in their New York apartment building.

I enjoyed my youth with a great deal of abandon. How much of this was mood disorder I could not tell you. As a single person I didn't notice; I just rode the waves of emotional highs and lows and didn't think much about it. I was an old pro at this by the time I was nineteen and met my husband. It was only through my association with him that I came to terms with my mood problems, although right before I met him I had checked myself in at a mental health clinic complaining that I sometimes felt unable to concentrate on one thing at a time.

I think I was twenty-two years old when my troubles cropped up again. At one point my husband and I went to see a psychologist. We talked about my mood swings and spells of nervousness, anger, and depression. The tiniest negative thing happening would cause long-lasting rage, very hard to quell. We told the psychologist of my father's history, even longer and grislier by then. He must have been in every state mental institution along the East coast. My grandmother, his mother, was wasting away by this time, losing her lifelong battle with chronic depression. I don't know much about her case except that she was chronically sad and starved herself to death after her husband passed away.

This man said my husband and I needed to lose weight; that was the extent of his advice. We did not see him much longer. By this time I was experiencing most of the symptoms I have today, although they have strengthened year by year. Sometimes I feel elated, exhilarated, with a great deal of energy. It sounds great, but you can get to be feeling so good that you scare the people around you, believe me! This is accompanied by light sleeping and nocturnal habits. I tend to become angry or aggressive when it is not appropriate, or just talk too loud. I often have a low self-image or feel sad. I sometimes have a hard time getting up to work, a heaviness that keeps me from moving. I get racing thoughts that make concentration hard. I have strong emotions that change rapidly. I tend to be physically clumsy. I develop unexplained skin rashes and sometimes feel like I'm generating electricity and shooting it out my fingers and toes. My judgment is often poor.

It was in my early twenties that I first used the herb cannabis for my condition. I had been exposed to it several times, the first when I was quite young. My mother had taken me to a mental health center after my initial signs of trouble as a child. After a group therapy session there some of the other kids took me riding and gave me a joint. Nothing at all happened, and I concluded it must be a mild drug.

When I was exposed to it later, I would actually choose it over alcohol because it didn't have such strong and negative effects on me. This is how I discovered that it was effective against most of my symptoms. Suppose I am in a fit of manic rage—the most destructive behavior of all. A few puffs of this herb and I can be calm. My husband and I have both noticed this; it is quite dramatic. One minute out of control in a mad rage over a meaningless detail, seemingly in need of a straitjacket, and somewhere, deep in my mind, asking myself why this is happening and why I can't get a handle on my own emotions. Then, within a few minutes, the time it takes to smoke a few pinches—why, I could even, after a round of apologies, laugh at myself!

But this herb is illegal, and I have a strong desire to abide by the law. My father was having great success with a new drug, lithium carbonate. I saw my father's physician, and he recommended that I try it. I took lithium for six months and experienced several adverse side effects—shaking, skin rashes, and loss of control over my speech. But I would still be taking it if it had worked for me as it did for my father. It literally restored his life. I had gotten worse, if anything.

The combination of lithium side effects and increased manic depressive symptoms drove me back to the use of cannabis. Some years later I tried to go without it again, this time because of increased social pressure against illegal drug use. It was a very difficult time for my family. Whenever I started to become manic, my husband and son would get scared and cower, triggering rage and making matters worse. When depression struck it was a black funk on our household. And I can tell you from the experience with my father, this can really destroy a family. After a while the knowledge that a little bit of herb would help me so much became irresistible. At first I tried eating cannabis but soon returned to smoking because I could control the dose better.

The legal situation now is worse than ever. I jeopardize my freedom and property in order to control my condition. Do I have a choice? I don't at all consider myself a drug abuser. I am doing what any rational person in my position would do. Cannabis does not cure my condition, and over the years it has probably continued to worsen. But with judicious use of this medicine my life is fine. I can control things with this drug that seems so harmless compared to the others I've tried, including tranquilizers as well as lithium. I am constantly concerned that I will be cut off from my supply of marihuana or caught with it in my possession. I feel my sanity may depend on it. Cannabis lessens what is troubling me and returns me to a more normal state. Often I do not experience a "high" at all, just a return to normal.

Here is the account of another woman who suffers from bipolar disorder and finds cannabis more useful than conventional medications:

I am a thirty-five-year-old woman with severe manic depression. When I was growing up I was hypersensitive, cried all the time, and fought with my brothers and sister. My parents always said they had to handle me with kid gloves. I had more energy than most and used it to the hilt. I was an agile gymnast and one of the fastest swimmers in my school. I was also at the top of my class in algebra and good at art and creative writing. I used to stay awake at night and dream up stories.

Around age fourteen my mood swings began to get more intense. I was agitated, restless, and constantly fighting at home. I lay awake at night and lost a lot of weight. Eventually I snapped and was sent to a mental hospital, where I was diagnosed as having manic-depressive disorder. They put me on lithium and told me I would have to take it the rest of my life. But lithium made me lethargic. I had trouble communicating and lost all my animation and creativity. Eventually I quit taking it. Recently I have also tried Tegretol [carbamazepine] and Depakote [valproic acid], neither of which helped. Tegretol started a manic episode, and Depakote had some very bad side effects. I'd like to find something else, but I don't have health insurance or the money to spend trying out new medications.

Since the age of fourteen I have had manic episodes regularly about once every six months. It would always start with not being able to sleep or eat. After two weeks I would just break down and seem to trip out into another world. Usually I ended up in a mental hospital.

I smoked marihuana for the first time in high school and couldn't believe how good it made me feel. My normally chaotic emotions subsided, and I had a sudden sense of calm, peace, and well-being. My perceptions of others and life changed dramatically. The world no longer seemed hostile but more within my control. I could sleep easily and actually had cravings for food. There were practically no side effects. When I had enough marihuana I would just naturally stop, because once you've gotten a certain effect you really don't want any more.

Only another manic-depressive using marihuana could possibly know how much this has changed the quality of my life. Although they don't know it, my family actually like me better when I'm stoned than when I'm taking lithium or not taking anything. When I'm stoned they can predict my moods and actually get close to me. But I can't tell my family or the doctors because it's illegal. I have to live a double life to get along.

I've often tried to quit marihuana, but I have a manic episode every time. Last year I decided I could control my emotional ups and downs without marihuana, but it led to one of the worst episodes I've ever experienced. I had been having trouble sleeping as usual. I began to get super clear vision that a disastrous earthquake was going to hit Los Angeles. I was feeling so good I was sure I was right. Soon I had my roommate convinced that we didn't have much time and would have to buy as many supplies as possible and then leave. We thought that after the quake the New World Order would be implemented and everyone would have to take the number that Revelations talks about in the Bible. We planned to go to El Salvador, where her family lives, and hide out for the next three and a half years. Crazy! But I really believed it. I maxed out all my credit cards, quit my job, and packed up all my things, including disguises I thought we were going to need. Eventually I had to return home with no job and major bills.

I knew then and there that I would have to go back on marihuana. It's been seven months now since I resumed smoking
marihuana, and I don't know what else to do. I have to choose
between obeying the law and staying sick or breaking the law
and being well.

Jacci Papi is a forty-five-year-old health professional and the mother
of a twenty-year-old son:

In late 1994 and early 1995 my son, Michael, age eighteen, began
to go out of control. He was unable to sleep, attend school, or
function in a normal fashion. He was running around nonstop,
acting on impulse without any sense of normal judgment. He
was in serious danger of accidentally harming himself or others.
There was no way to reason with him, because he was unable to
think or listen long enough to understand what you were trying
to say. He had become a human time-bomb.

Then, on February 14, 1995, he had a full-blown psychotic
manic episode and refused treatment. I had to petition a court
to commit him to a psychiatric hospital, where he was given a
diagnosis of manic-depressive disorder. Both Michael's father and
my grandmother suffered from the same disorder, which is now
called bipolar disorder.

During his nine days in the hospital (the time allotted by my
insurance company) Michael was given lithium and Trilafon [per-
phenazine, an antipsychotic drug]. We were told that he would
need lithium for the rest of his life. They explained that it worked
very well in 60 percent of people with this disorder.

We returned home, and for the first month or two, the mania
seemed to have ended. At the end of the second month the Trilafon was discontinued, but Michael was still taking a high dose
of lithium. At that point he developed a rash on his neck and
chest; he also had dark circles under his eyes and was incoherent
most of the time. The lithium level in his blood was exactly
where the doctor wanted it, but now he was acting like an Alzheimer's patient. He couldn't read or comprehend a paragraph,
let alone finish school. He was detached from his surrounding

and himself. There was no emotional content left in him. He was becoming unrecognizable. He had always been very much like Robin Williams in personality and extremely athletic—a skier, football player, and weight lifter. It was heartbreaking to watch him lose himself in a medicated stupor. I became convinced that lithium did not eliminate the disease but instead was drowning his brain so the symptoms could not be activated. I could still see tiny mood swings and moments of complete restlessness, but in a body that was unable to become hypomanic.

Michael decided to cut his lithium in half. I knew this would be dangerous but I agreed that something had to be done. Soon he was more himself, laughing and talking and almost back among the living. Then he started to become more hypomanic, and I knew we were headed for trouble. He was back to the energy level of someone on high doses of speed, and this lasted for months. He was running through life like a high-bred stallion, while I was gathering everything ever written on manic-depressive disorder.

Then one day he came home and was perfectly normal in every respect. I thought that maybe he was in remission because the disease is known to do that, and I was thrilled at the possibility. Later that night he was back to full speed ahead, and all hope sank within me. This continued as the weeks passed. There would be times when he was perfectly normal, but only for short intervals. I could not figure it out. I started to chart his sleep pattern, his food intake, the kinds of foods, what chemicals he was subjecting himself to, and so on. Finally I discovered that he was smoking pot. Of course I freaked out. We talked about it at length and he told me point blank, "I only feel normal when I smoke a joint." By this time I was ready to blame the disease on his pot smoking. I was totally irrational about this. Michael and I fought constantly for a month about it. Finally he asked me to research cannabis and let him know what I found. I figured I would be able to find enough damaging information to put the subject to rest. The next week was my week of discovery. Not only could I not find what I was looking for, but I became convinced that there was no permanent damage and that cannabis was actually helpful for people with mood disorders.

I went on-line on the computer to talk to other people suffering from bipolar disorder, and I was overwhelmed by the first-person stories of the benefits others had found.

The hardest part of this entire thing was rearranging my value system. I was raised to be a law-abiding citizen. Although I grew up in the 1960s and had tried pot and inhaled, I was never a regular user because it was illegal. I raised Mike right. He was taught to respect his elders, do what you are supposed to do, and above all follow the law.

It is hard enough to live with an eighteen-year-old during a naturally rebellious time, but to be forced to participate in an illegal activity is the absolute worst scenario. But that is exactly what I'm doing. Mike has been smoking pot for two months now. He does not smoke daily, but when the mania begins he smokes and within five minutes he is fine. He never appears to be "high," just happy and relaxed. We don't have to deal with mood swings anymore. He can work on his home-schooling program, and I don't doubt that he will finish by the end of summer. He has been repairing lobster traps with a friend and will be lobstering six days a week by the end of April.

At this point I expect to be arrested some day, because if Mike gets arrested, they will have to take me right along with him. I plan to grow a plant this summer for his use. I know I could end up in jail, but I also know that without some kind of medication that works, my son could end up in jail, institutionalized, or dead. What choice do I have?

Except for the eight Americans who have Compassionate INDs, every one of the many thousands who use marihuana as a medicine runs a risk of being arrested. They have to worry about financial ruin, loss of their careers, and forfeiture of their automobiles and homes. Some have an additional burden, because mandatory school drug programs and Parents for a Drug-Free America advertisements have

given their children an exaggerated idea of the dangers of using marihuana. Many of these children become concerned about the health
and well-being of their marihuana-using parents. A few of those parents have been arrested because their worried children informed on
them to the police officers who serve as instructors in the popular
school drug program known as Drug Abuse Resistance Education
(DARE). The following accounts are by a forty-year-old software engineer and his thirty-seven-year-old wife, who suffers from bipolar disorder. He speaks first:

My wife and I and our two boys live in Tyngsboro, Massachusetts.
My wife was given a diagnosis of bipolar disorder in 1982 and
has been taking lithium since 1992. She also uses marihuana for
her symptoms. She has had six psychiatrists in the past fourteen
years and has been interviewed by many more. I have always told
them that she uses marihuana regularly, and not one of them has
told her to stop. They do not even seem to care or pay attention.

I posted a question about this to the alt.support.depression.
manic newsgroup on the Internet. I asked whether doctors knew
something about marihuana but could not recommend it because
of its illegality. The responses were varied, but most people who
were manic-depressive said that marihuana helped them, and
one said that some doctors considered it effective in controlling
mood disorders.

My wife functions much better when she uses marihuana.
When she is hypomanic, it relaxes her, helps her sleep, and slows
her speech down. When she is depressed and would otherwise lie
in bed all day, the marihuana makes her more active. When she
runs out of marihuana and can't get more, she becomes more irritable and hard to live with. Lithium is also effective, but it doesn't
always keep her in control during seasonal mood changes.

Our dilemma is that our thirteen-year-old has been through
the DARE program and has learned about the evils of drugs and
alcohol. He opposes all substance use, legal or illegal — and I want
it that way. But he knows that my wife uses marihuana, and it

"eats" at him, although he also knows about her illness and how marihuana helps. Understandably, all this confuses him.

I believe that marihuana could help some people if it were made available as a prescription medicine. Certainly there are other health and social issues involved, and I can't decide what would be right for the country as a whole. All I know is that in this family it has relieved us all of much suffering.

Now his wife:

I am thirty-seven, and I have been using marihuana for twenty years. I was diagnosed bipolar in 1982. I take lithium and Wellbutrin [bupropion], although I dislike these drugs. I've gained about forty pounds since I started taking lithium, but otherwise there are no side effects.

My thirteen-year-old son knows about my illness. He has also known about my marihuana smoking for about five years. He realized what I was doing after he participated in the DARE program in school. It bothers me when he comes home and says they talked about drugs and he was thinking that his mother is "one of them." He doesn't want anyone to know his mother is a "druggie," and until now we've kept it our secret. I don't think he would tell anyone, but I'm still afraid something might get out. Sometimes these programs use tricks to get kids to inform on their friends and relatives. They say, "If you really care about this person, the only way you can help them is to report them."

My husband has talked to him about it. He has explained that lithium and the other medications I'm taking are drugs. He also explained that many legal drugs are far more dangerous than marihuana and that no one has ever died from using marihuana. But my son insists that if it is illegal, then it is wrong. This bothers me so much that I have considered stopping.

The trouble is that at times when I feel tired and run-down, just a couple puffs of marihuana bring me back to life. Sometimes I think it brings me to a level of normalcy that everyone else achieves naturally. At other times, when everything seems to be going like a whirlwind around me and I can't keep track of what I'm thinking about or saying or feeling, the marihuana just seems to slow the world down a bit. When I have trouble sleeping, it helps zonk me out, but if I have trouble waking up it brings me to life. I don't like being thought of as a "drug-abusing mother," but I actually think I'm a better mom when I'm feeling in control because of marihuana.

Here is another account of cannabis use by a person with bipolar disorder, emphasizing the reduction of lithium side effects:

I am twenty-nine years old, born and raised in North Carolina. My academic background is in English literature, computer science, and law; I now work as a technology consultant and writer, although I am contemplating returning to graduate school. I am divorced. I am reasonably active in my community, though work takes much of my time these days.

I was first diagnosed with bipolar disorder about five years ago, when I was in law school (a psychiatrist also tentatively ventured this diagnosis during my undergraduate years), but I suspect that I have had a mood disorder for most of my life. I was certainly clinically depressed as early as age nine, and my first hypomanic episode occurred at seventeen. There is also a family history of mood disorders, especially on my mother's side. All three of her brothers had "mercurial" personalities, and they all experienced tremendous successes and notable failures in business. Their extravagance and outgoing personalities resemble my behavior while manic or hypomanic. Although none of them was formally diagnosed with a mood disorder, both my parents have been treated for clinical depression.

Before I was diagnosed and found the right treatment, I had the typical symptoms of bipolar disorder. During depressive phases I became withdrawn, uncommunicative, and preoccupied with suicide. I found it nearly impossible to function in school or at work. During hypomanic or manic phases I spent freely, traveled all over the country (and world), made poor personal and business decisions, engaged in risky sexual behavior, and so forth. The illness has caused me a great deal of personal pain as well as financial woes. I separated from my wife (who eventually divorced me) the summer before I was diagnosed. I've lost jobs, ruined friendships, and alienated members of my family. Fortunately, much of this damage has been repaired with time and understanding. I thank God that my ruined credit rating is the only apparent lasting harm.

Thanks to lithium and sensible therapy, including the judicious use of cannabis, I have been relatively stable and sane for the past three years, although my sleep is often disturbed and I still have (very much milder) hypomania and depression in much the same cyclic pattern as before.

I first used cannabis in my freshman year of college (1984). I preferred it to alcohol as an intoxicant and used it a few times a week, almost always by smoking (I still prefer to take it that way). In retrospect, it seems clear to me that I was medicating myself for bipolar disorder even then. When depressed and anxious, I found that cannabis was soothing and enhanced my ability to enjoy life. When I was in a manic phase, it relaxed me and helped me get to sleep. I often felt as though I had so much energy inside me that I would jump out of my skin; the cannabis helped tremendously with that. But there was a downside. Manics have a big problem with impulse control, and cannabis seemed to exacerbate it. ("Drive to Canada? Great idea. Let's go!") It also ratcheted up my already overactive libido a notch or two, which wasn't the healthiest thing in the world.

When I was diagnosed and began treatment with lithium, I got almost immediate relief, but I also suffered from nausea, pounding headaches, hand tremors, and excess production of saliva. A friend suggested that I try getting high, reasoning that if cannabis helped chemotherapy patients deal with their nausea and discomfort, it might help me too. My doctors thought the idea was absurd but admitted that it would be safe to take cannabis together with lithium. So I tried it, and the results were remarkable. The hand tremors subsided, the headaches vanished, and the saliva factory resumed normal production levels. All I needed was one or two puffs on a marihuana cigarette. When lithium side effects get bad, the availability of cannabis has been an absolute godsend. It is also nice to be able to use cannabis as an intoxicant, knowing that, unlike the combination of lithium and alcohol, it cannot damage my kidneys.

Bipolar disorder is naturally cyclical; manic and depressive episodes come and go, so it is essential not to confuse natural remission with cannabis-induced improvement. And of course, the proportion of patients with mood disorders who would get the kinds of benefits described here is unknown. As usual, promising anecdotal evidence points to the need for more systematic clinical investigation.

3 Less Common Medical Uses

Although almost all the evidence of marihuana's medical usefulness is anecdotal, in the case of certain disorders it appears to be
firmly established. In the treatment of the nausea and vomiting of
cancer chemotherapy, glaucoma, epilepsy, the muscle spasms of
multiple sclerosis, paraplegia, and quadriplegia, the nausea and
weight-loss syndrome of AIDS, chronic pain, migraine, pruritus,
menstrual cramps, labor pains, and depression and other mood
disorders, so many patients have used cannabis successfully that
it is difficult to believe that the palliative effects are not real and
reliable. It is inconceivable that all these patients are reporting
merely placebo effects or some shared delusion.

Other medical uses of cannabis are reported less often. One
reason is that the exploration of medical cannabis is only beginning as the knowledge of its uses becomes more widely accepted.
Another reason is that some of the symptoms and syndromes for
which cannabis may be useful are rare; it takes time for knowledge of its therapeutic value to spread among people suffering
from these uncommon disorders. Furthermore, sometimes only
a small proportion of people suffering from a particular disorder
find cannabis useful. And of course the placebo effect is as real
for cannabis as for any other medicine.

The following medical uses of cannabis are more speculative
than those described in the previous chapter, but there is reason
to believe they will eventually be accepted.

ASTHMA

About 10 million Americans suffer from asthma—attacks of breathlessness and wheezing caused by narrowing of the bronchioles, small airways in the lungs. The linings of the bronchioles become inflamed and swollen, and fill with phlegm; a chronic cough may develop from attempts to free the obstruction. Asthma attacks kill more than 4,000 Americans each year. The disorder is caused by allergic reactions to pollen, dust, feathers, and animal hair, and also by cold air, infections, exercise, and air pollutants. It is more common in children than adults and usually grows less severe with age. Bronchodilators can be used to relax the bronchial muscles and widen the airway; synthetic steroids reduce inflammation and the resulting swelling. But beta-agonists, the drugs most commonly used as bronchodilators, may cause sleeplessness, jitteriness, and nausea; and steroids, when used for more than a few months, have more serious side effects, including bone loss, seizures, and bleeding. (These can be mitigated somewhat if an inhaler is used to deliver the steroid directly to the lungs, without passage through the bloodstream.) Other anti-inflammatory drugs also have serious side effects and are more difficult to administer.

Given the limitations of existing drugs in the treatment of asthma, the use of cannabinoids should be considered. Several studies have shown that THC acts as a bronchodilator in both normal subjects and patients with either chronic bronchial asthma or experimentally induced bronchial spasms. In one study, THC allowed a freer flow of air in and out of the lungs of healthy subjects; in asthmatic patients, it reversed bronchial constriction. In a related study, smoked THC was compared with inhaled isoproterenol, a standard bronchodilator. Both drugs relieved bronchial spasms; isoproterenol worked faster and had a stronger peak effect, but the effect of THC lasted longer.[1]

1. D. P. Tashkin, B. J. Shapiro, and I. A. Frank, "Acute Pulmonary Physiologic Effects of Smoked Marihuana and Oral Delta-9-tetrahydrocannabinol in Healthy Young Men," *New England Journal of Medicine* 289 (1973): 336–341; D. P. Tashkin, B. J. Shapiro, Y. E. Lee, and C. E. Harper, "Effects of Smoked Marihuana in Experimentally Induced Asthma," *American Review of Respiratory Disease* 112 (1975): 377–386.

Whole marihuana is probably not generally useful for this purpose because the irritating effects of THC and the tars in marihuana smoke have the potential to produce chronic bronchitis in heavy users. Cannabis smoke also contains carcinogens and substances that are toxic to the cilia, hairlike cells that help free the lungs of mucus.

The alternatives to smoking are oral use and spray inhalers. But the anti-asthmatic activity of oral THC is delayed and unreliable because of its erratic absorption. When THC is delivered as an aerosol spray, some experiments have found significant dilation of the bronchi without adverse effects. In one experiment, THC in aerosol form produced a faster but shorter-acting effect than the standard bronchodilator, isoproterenol.[2] This line of research has not been pursued because THC in spray form is still a bronchial irritant.[3] Nevertheless, there are compelling reasons to continue research. Other cannabinoids, natural or synthetic, may prove to be more effective than THC or to have fewer side effects. Safer ways of delivering these drugs may be discovered. Finally, the mechanism of action of cannabinoids is apparently different from that of other bronchodilators, and new treatments may be developed if that mechanism can be identified. The need for new approaches is indicated by a study demonstrating that the use of beta-agonist bronchodilators is riskier than previously believed, and in fact is associated with high death rates in asthma sufferers.[4]

The following is an account by a forty-three-year-old software engineer who has suffered from asthma since he was three years old:

My first treatment was a cocktail containing mainly ephedrine, theophylline, and phenobarbital, which I took for a couple of decades. Ephedrine is a stimulant that activates the adrenaline

2. L. Vachon, A. Robins, and E. A. Gaensler, "Airways Response to Aerosolized Delta-9-tetrahydrocannabinol: Preliminary Report," in *The Therapeutic Potential of Marijuana,* ed. S. Cohen and R. C. Stillman (New York: Plenum, 1976).

3. D. P. Tashkin, S. Reiss, B. J. Shapiro, B. Calvarese, J. L. Olson, and J. W. Lodge, "Bronchial Effects of Aerosolized Delta-9-THC in Healthy and Asthmatic Subjects," *American Review of Respiratory Disease* 115 (1977): 57–65.

4. W. O. Spitzer, S. Suissa, P. Ernst, et al., "The Use of Beta-agonists and the Risk of Death and Near Death from Asthma," *New England Journal of Medicine* 326 (1992): 501–506.

system and helps relieve asthma by opening the airways. Unfortunately, it causes nervousness and insomnia, and tolerance develops after a few days. It can also aggravate the toxic effects of other anti-asthma stimulants, including theophylline. Phenobarbital is added to counter the jitters and insomnia caused by stimulants, but you can't take too high a dose, since asthma often worsens during the night and it is better not to be in a drugged sleep when that happens.

Most of my friends in college used marihuana regularly, but I avoided it because I was afraid it would make my lungs even worse. Fear of the law was also a concern, since one of my friends was arrested three times for possession and served four weekends in jail. A friend from church, a retired jazz musician, told me he had smoked marihuana for thirty years. He quit without difficulty when he decided that the police had learned to recognize it. He didn't think marihuana was dangerous, but he advised young people not to use it because of the law.

When I graduated from college, I applied to the Peace Corps but was rejected because of my asthma. Eventually I got a job with the federal government and moved to Washington. Working in a stuffy federal office building full of smokers was no fun. My sinuses ran and my throat burned, and by the end of the day I was panting for breath. I tried various doses and combinations of anti-asthma drugs, mainly theophylline, but I was always left panting in my smoke-filled office, and I didn't sleep well. The prescribed dose was insufficient during the day and too much at night.

In college I began cycling for fun and transportation. It seemed to make my breathing easier, and soon I found I could take long bicycle trips. I still cycle five thousand miles a year. I complained about my problem to a cyclist friend who also has asthma, and she told me she just smokes some marihuana when she starts wheezing. I tried it, but the smoke was irritating and the relief was temporary. The wheezing would soon return and seemed worse than before. Then I remembered from the Peter Sellers movie *I Love You, Alice B. Toklas* that you could bake marihuana in cookies, so I tried that and found that it gave me rapid and effective relief without a rebound effect. It also seemed to make the anti-asthmatic stimulants work better. I explained this to my doctor, and he gave me permission to use marihuana.

For several years oral marihuana provided a relaxing alternative to the constant use of theophylline and isoproterenol. When my asthma flared up, marihuana was so effective that I could tolerate a smoke-filled room. I don't get that level of relief from my normal medications. I experimented and found that a half ounce baked in cookies would make fifty to one hundred doses, each lasting eight to sixteen hours. Relief would come in a half hour to one hour.

My marihuana use had at least one effect on my career. In 1981 I began to work with computers, which luckily meant that I was able to spend much of my time in rooms where smoking was prohibited. I applied for a job and was asked to list all the organizations to which I had ever belonged. I answered honestly that I belonged to NORML [National Organization for the Reform of Marijuana Laws]. They asked me to explain my marihuana use and told me that I couldn't get a security clearance if I had used it in the past five years. One of my supervisors learned about this and hinted that my job was in danger, so I resigned and found another job doing unclassified work.

INSOMNIA

Cannabis has a long history as a hypnotic (sleep-inducing) drug, and many people use it for that purpose today, including one of the multiple sclerosis patients and several of the bipolar patients who tell their stories here. There is now experimental evidence that the hypnotic effects are produced by cannabidiol rather than THC. One controlled study of fifteen insomniac patients found that over a five-week period "sleep quality was significantly influenced by 160 mg of cannabidiol as two-thirds of the subjects slept more than seven hours. . . . Most subjects had few interruptions of sleep and reported having a good night's sleep."[5] Legally available hypnotics leave much to be desired. Tolerance develops to most of them, many cause rebound insomnia, some are addictive, and all have the potential for a lethal overdose. Given these drawbacks, it is unfortunate that the hypnotic potential of cannabis in general and of cannabidiol in particular has not been more thoroughly explored.

OTHER CAUSES OF SEVERE NAUSEA

Cancer and AIDS patients are not the only ones who can make use of marihuana's antinauseant and appetite-stimulating effects. It has also been used by women who suffer from the rare disorder known as hyperemesis gravidarum—a greatly heightened form of morning sickness in which the sufferer has nearly constant nausea and vomiting throughout pregnancy. In the past, abortion was sometimes necessary to save the woman's life. More recently these women have been hospitalized and fed intravenously. Some have now discovered that they can smoke marihuana daily instead—a practice that probably poses less risk to the fetus than the alternatives of prolonged intravenous feeding or standard antiemetic drugs.

Kidney failure is another potential cause of severe nausea. The following account is by James C. Longcope, M.D., a psychiatrist:

> George Duborg was hospitalized in September 1991 with all the symptoms of major depression. He slept in two-hour snatches. He lacked appetite and energy and had lost fifty to sixty pounds in two months. He was irritable, and his concentration was poor. He had not been able to distract himself by reading for several weeks, and although he was a baseball fan, he could not even muster any interest in the World Series. Although he was not suicidal, he said he wished "someone would put me out of my misery."
>
> At age sixty-two George was a successful investment broker

5. E. A. Carlini and J. M. Cunha, "Hypnotic and Antiepileptic Effects of Cannabidiol," *Journal of Clinical Pharmacology* 21 (1981): 417S–427S.

with a stable marriage and healthy children, all of them out of college and making their way in the world. But he had a lot to be depressed about, since he had lost the function of his kidneys. Several months before the hospitalization he had taken a non-steroidal anti-inflammatory agent for intractable migraine head-aches. It caused partial kidney failure, which became total kidney failure after an idiosyncratic reaction to an intravenous diagnostic procedure. He was being sustained by renal dialysis as he waited for a kidney donor.

But George's problem was not just renal failure or depression. It was a symptom that had become more devastating than his disease: nausea. Spasms of nausea and hiccoughs waxed and waned but never went away. The dialysis was adjusted and minor electrolyte imbalances were corrected, but the nausea persisted. Compazine did not help. Zantac did not help. Zofran, a widely heralded new intravenous antinausea drug, did not help, even when given every two hours. The antidepressant nortriptyline had to be discontinued because of liver toxicity. When I introduced myself, George said, "I don't need a psychiatrist. I need something for this terrible nausea. I will deal with my depression and my fate if you give me a level playing field."

His internist had ordered Marinol, and the hospital pharmacy was trying to obtain it. Although he was willing to try anything, we decided to wait for the Marinol. On October 19 it arrived, and George received three 5 mg doses in the next twenty-four hours. On October 20 I stopped by to see how he was doing. "See, I told you," he said, "give me a level playing field and I will manage my fate." He was playing gin with his wife and invited me to join. "We would be glad to have your company until the World Series comes on; just don't pull any psychiatrist tricks. I'm doing fine; this stuff works. I can barely remember how bad I was." It was like finding Sam Magee "sitting cool and calm in the heart of the furnace roar." George needed Marinol again in the next three days, and then went twenty-four hours without it. The nausea and hiccoughs came and went several times over the next few weeks, and each time 5–10 mg of Marinol controlled the symptoms.

Today George is alive and well. Because his kidney function recovered spontaneously, he was able to discontinue dialysis. Even the migraine headaches have improved, or at least don't seem quite as bad. Tetrahydrocannabinol had helped him through the worst phase when nothing else worked.

Marihuana in its natural form can be useful for patients with chronic renal failure, as this account by Murphy Canter indicates:

I am twenty-five and have had severe kidney disease for many years. When I was fifteen my mother donated her kidney for a transplant, but it failed five years later. My sister provided a second transplant, but it failed after three more years. In February 1993 I went on a kidney dialysis regimen of three weekly three-and-a-half-hour treatments. It kept me constantly nauseated and made eating difficult. After five months my weight fell from 190 pounds to 120 pounds (I am six feet tall). I took Compazine [prochlorperazine] for the nausea, but it had a zombifying effect.

I already knew about the medical effects of cannabis. Because of the transplants I had to take prednisone [a steroid], cyclosporine [an immune system suppressant], and Imuran [azathioprine, another anti-immune drug]. Cyclosporine caused nausea, heartburn, and insomnia. Prednisone and Imuran caused digestive-tract pain, nausea, mood swings, nightmares, and acne. The doctors prescribed many drugs to counteract these side effects, but none of them worked. Cannabis was the only substance that allowed me to feel human enough to attend high school and college.

So in June 1993 I turned to a medicine that I knew would be effective. I began to smoke it regularly, and now I take it with a doctor's approval. The only other medications I take are erythromycin [an antibiotic] and Phos-Lo [a calcium supplement]. I smoke marihuana before meals to stimulate my appetite and after meals to prevent nausea and vomiting. Now I weigh 150 pounds, and I give cannabis the credit. It relieves my nausea better than any other substance I have ever used.

Cannabis is also the first drug that has been effective in controlling my high blood pressure. I have taken so many others that I can't remember their names, but the result was always the same: they either didn't work or caused such horrible side effects that I needed more drugs, which only raised my blood pressure again. Since I began smoking cannabis, my blood pressure has remained relatively constant at 130 over 80.

Marihuana also relieves mild pain from cramps or headaches. Being in dialysis means having the equivalent of a knitting needle stuck into your vein six times a week. I also get terrible cramps in my legs and arms, and I have been through surgery under general anesthesia over twenty times. Cannabis relieves my pain faster and for a longer time than Tylenol, Advil, or aspirin, without upsetting an already queasy stomach.

There are psychological benefits, too. I have a tendency toward depression, and I suffer terrible anxiety attacks on dialysis days as the hour draws near. Marihuana allows me to tolerate the situation and put most of the blackness in the back of my mind.

Unfortunately, there are some serious problems, none of which has anything to do with the effects of marihuana itself. The price is staggering, since insurance will not pay for it. It is far more expensive than any prescription medicine. And buying it can be dangerous if not impossible. I have to put myself at great risk to save my own life. Can you imagine a postoperative patient asking for morphine for pain relief and having a nurse say, "Well, the guy wasn't home and I think he has to work until ten. Call me tomorrow and I'll see if I can score any from the hospital next door." Finally, the quality of marihuana is chancy. If only a low grade is available, I have to inhale more, and this can cause bronchitis.

I won't get over these problems until the politics changes. The present official word is that marihuana is not medicine. We need a new word from people like myself who have been made experts by nature: marihuana is medicine and can save lives.

ANTIMICROBIAL EFFECTS

Another possible medical use of cannabis is suggested by the work of some investigators at Palacky University in Olomouc, Czechoslovakia. They found that cannabis extracts containing cannabidiolic acid produce impressive antibacterial effects on a number of microorganisms, including strains of staphylococcus that resist penicillin and other antibiotics. They successfully treated a variety of conditions, including ear infections, with cannabis lotions and ointments. Topical application of cannabis relieved pain and prevented infection in second-degree burns. The Czech researchers report that a pathologist injured his thumb in the dissecting room and the resulting infection resisted all available treatments. Amputation was being considered when a cannabis extract overcame the infection. If these findings are confirmed, they may prove especially important at a time when so many bacterial strains have become resistant to antibiotics.[6]

Cannabis may also be useful for the symptomatic relief of herpes, a viral disease. People who suffer cold sores or genital herpes have steeped marihuana in rubbing alcohol until the solution turns greenish and dabbed it on the site of an imminent herpetic-sore outbreak. They say it prevents blistering and makes the sores disappear in a day or two. So far these reports are only anecdotal, but they are certainly worth following up. There is now some evidence that THC actually binds to the herpes virus and inactivates it.[7]

6. J. Kabelik, Z. Krejci, and F. Santavy, "Cannabis as a Medicament," *Bulletin of Narcotics* 12 (1960): 20–22; Z. Krejci, "On the Problem of Substances with Antibacterial Action: Cannabis Effect," *Casopis Lekaru Ceskych* 43 (1961): 1351–1354.

7. G. Lancz, S. Specter, H. K. Brown, J. F. Hackney, and H. Friedman, "Interaction of Delta-9-tetrahydrocannabinol with Herpes Viruses and Cultural Conditions Associated with Drug-induced Anti-cellular Effects," in *Drugs of Abuse, Immunity, and Immunodeficiency*, ed. H. Friedman, et al. (New York: Plenum, 1991), 278–304; G. Lancz, S. Specter, and H. K. Brown, "Suppressive Effect of Delta-9-tetrahydrocannabinol on Herpes Simplex Virus Infectivity in Vitro," *Proceedings of the Society for Experimental Biology and Medicine* 196 (1991): 401–404.

TOPICAL ANESTHETIC EFFECTS

A hundred years ago physicians knew that cannabis was an effective topical anesthetic, especially for the mucous membranes of the mouth and tongue. Dentists of that era used it in the form of a tincture of cannabis in alcohol. Although modern dentists show little interest, some patients have now rediscovered it. A fifty-two-year-old woman describes this use of cannabis as follows:

> The bones under my lower gums are disintegrating as my mother's did. About twelve years ago I had "flap" surgery: the dentist cleaned all the particles of bone, etc., out. Ever since I have been losing my lower teeth, and my gums are chronically agitated. A couple of months ago a friend put a few drops of tincture of cannabis under my tongue to help me sleep. It burned, but not unpleasantly, as it rolled over my mouth. To my amazement, my gums did not hurt at all for two or three days afterward. I wish it were not so hard to get this wonderful medicine.

ANTITUMORAL EFFECTS

The relief of nausea and vomiting in chemotherapy is not the only proposed use of cannabis in cancer treatment. In the 1970s an experiment was conducted in which the lungs of mice were injected with cancer cells, and delta-9-THC, delta-8-THC, or cannabinol was applied; the size of the tumors dropped 25 to 82 percent, depending on dose and duration of treatment, with a corresponding increase in survival time.[8] Other animal studies also suggest that some cannabinoids have tumor-reducing properties. Although there is no human and little other research in this field, cannabinoids might prove to be useful as adjuncts to other chemotherapeutic agents.

8. L. S. Harris, A. E. Munson, and R. A. Carchman, "Antitumor Properties of Cannabinoids," in *The Pharmacology of Marihuana,* ed. M. C. Braude and S. Szara, 2 vols. (New York: Raven, 1976), 2:773–776.

DYSTONIAS

Dystonia is a neurological syndrome consisting of involuntary sustained (tonic) or spasmodic (clonic) muscle contractions. It often causes twisting and other abnormal movements or postures whose timing and intensity can be influenced by various factors, including stress, fatigue, and sleep. The most common form, which affects the neck, is known as cervical dystonia or spasmodic torticollis. Dystonia is distinguished from choreiform (writhing) and myoclonic (jerky) motions by its repetitive and patterned quality. Dystonia may be idiopathic (of unknown origin) or the result of various brain lesions, neurodegenerative disorders, and toxins. Standard medications are only sporadically effective and at best give short-term relief. Recently doctors have been testing botulinum toxin, which prevents contractions by blocking the nerve supply of the muscle and paralyzing it. But this treatment is expensive, and patients often develop immunity to the toxin.

The following account is by a sixty-two-year-old woman who suffers from spasmodic torticollis:

> It is almost ten years since I first became aware that something had gone awry in my body. I could not turn my head to the right without a great deal of pain and very strong tremors. I would awaken in the morning with no feeling at all in my left foot and leg as well as numbness in my left arm and hand. Co-workers noticed that my gait was strange. I was bumping into things because I could not always see to my right. I was also having respiratory problems. After many tests I was told that I had a severely compressed spinal cord and two herniated cervical discs.
>
> Surgery relieved the spinal cord compression, and I regained circulation on the left side of my body, but recuperation did not go well. My head, pulling constantly to the left, caused pain at the site of the incision on the front of my neck. Eventually a neurologist gave me the diagnosis of spasmodic torticollis.

In the years since, my appetite has often been poor and I have suffered from insomnia. I can no longer work as a college teacher because of the pain and fatigue. Social situations are often a nightmare. I usually wear a cervical collar to support my head. People stare at me in public, and I never know when I might emit an involuntary groan of pain or drop something when a muscle goes into a spasm.

I have tried many treatments, including physical therapy, biofeedback, acupressure and acupuncture, Chinese herbs, and many, many drugs. I don't remember them all, but I know that I was given Vicodin [hydrocodone and acetaminophen], Percodan [oxycodone and aspirin], fentanyl, methadone, Dilaudid [hydromorphone], and MS Contin [morphine] for the pain. For the muscle spasms I have taken Ativan [lorazepam], Valium [diazepam], Artane [trihexyphenidyl], Robaxin [methocarbamol], Soma [carisoprodol], and Dilantin [phenytoin]. For depression I have taken Desyrel [trazodone] and Prozac [fluoxetine]. I've even tried an experimental treatment—injection of botulinum toxin into the affected muscles to block the electrical impulses from the brain that cause the abnormal activity. The toxin had unpleasant side effects, including nausea, headaches, muscle pain, and weakness, and after eighteen months I developed resistance to it.

None of these drugs had much effect, and there were many times when they made me so ill I wished I would die. I am no longer taking any of them, although I go to a hospital periodically for steroid injections.

I have found that the most effective treatment is marihuana, which was first suggested to me by a doctor. It relaxes my spasms with no side effects except the fear of being arrested (I take it in cookies or tea because smoking irritates my throat and lungs). This natural substance is clearly superior to the synthetic drugs I used to take. I work with a support group for patients with dystonia and I know the suffering it causes. It is wrong to withhold anything that relieves the pain. Doctors are honor-bound to prevent suffering, and they need to question the position of the American Medical Association on the issue of medical marihuana.

Cannabidiol may be responsible for the antidystonic properties of marihuana, which have been noticed at least since 1981.[9] In one study cannabidiol was given, along with standard medications, to five patients with dystonic movement disorders. All improved 20 to 50 percent over a six-week period with few side effects.[10] As far as we know, this potential medical use of cannabis has not been explored further. Some of the neuroleptic drugs prescribed for patients with chronic psychotic disorders occasionally cause dystonias. The symptoms can be disfiguring and incapacitating, and present treatments are inadequate. Psychiatrists who must prescribe antipsychotic drugs might consider exploring the use of cannabidiol to counter this serious effect.

ADULT ATTENTION DEFICIT DISORDER

Attention deficit disorder (ADD) is best known as a childhood disorder, but it has become increasingly clear that it also occurs in adolescents and adults. Adults with ADD are impatient, restless, moody, insecure, and easily bored. They have trouble setting priorities, managing their time, meeting appointments, and keeping track of possessions. They often have brief, stormy love affairs, change jobs frequently, and fail to fulfill what they and others regard as their potential. Many of them suffer from anxiety or chronic mild depression. A large proportion develop alcoholism or other drug problems.

The following account is by a twenty-five-year-old student at California State University at Hayward who suffers from ADD and believes that without the help of cannabis he might not be able to graduate:

9. C. D. Marsden, "Treatment of Torsion Dystonia," in *Disorders of Movement: Current Status of Modern Therapy*, vol. 8, ed. A. Barbeau (Philadelphia: J. B. Lippincott, 1981), 81–104.

10. P. Consroe, R. Sandyk, and S. R. Snider, "Open Label Evaluation of Cannabidiol in Dystonic Movement Disorders," *International Journal of Neuroscience* 30 (1986): 277–282.

Ever since I was a little boy, teachers and other adults have said I was too energetic and active. When I was in middle school, my parents cut sugar and stimulants out of my diet. My teachers often said that if I paid more attention, applied myself, and focused on the task at hand I would have a promising future. Despite my habits I managed to make slightly above average grades and pass all my courses. But in college I saw that there was a difference between me and other students. I simply couldn't sit still for long periods of time; my thoughts and body desired to wander beyond the classroom.

At the end of my sophomore year I was tested at the University of California at Davis medical school and given a diagnosis of adult attention deficit disorder. My psychiatrist prescribed Cylert [pemoline, a stimulant] to bring my level of excitement down. For months I was to take three pills a day. Immediately after taking the pill I felt more excitement than ever, and then eventually my activity would decrease to a steady "normal" level. But this going up and coming down was uncomfortable, and there were also terrible side effects, my thoughts raced, my hands perspired, my heart pounded ferociously, and I couldn't sleep. I recall countless nights staring at my bedroom ceiling listening to my heart.

After six or seven months of this I tried a drug recommended by a friend at the University of California at Santa Cruz. She was an honor student who wrote for the school newspaper, and she said this drug relaxed the body while generating an active mind and enhancing creativity. It was cannabis, and it worked. I now smoke from a pipe three times a day, just as I used to take Cylert. I am more relaxed, I sleep much better, and I think and write more clearly. Ideas are flowing, and my studies have become more interesting. Cannabis allows me to think and analyze beyond the assignment. It eliminates the worried or anxious thoughts that used to interrupt my efforts to write, listen to lectures, or participate in serious conversations. As my ability to concentrate has improved, so have my grades. Ordinary distractions have lost their power to play havoc with my attention. I can center my efforts on the task at hand while fragmented thoughts fade into the background. Combining the use of cannabis with a written weekly schedule and many interpersonal relationships, I am able to negate the symptoms of ADD.

SCHIZOPHRENIA

The impact of cannabis on people with schizophrenia is disputed. It is sometimes thought to precipitate acute schizophrenic episodes, yet schizophrenic patients who use it generally regard it as helpful. In our experience, some of them find that it counteracts the undesirable effects of their antipsychotic medications without causing any problems of its own. In a study comparing schizophrenic patients who used cannabis with those who did not, researchers found no evidence that it made their symptoms worse or led to more relapses. On the contrary, patients who smoked marihuana had fewer delusions and, above all, fewer of the so-called negative symptoms, which include apathy, limited speech, and emotional unresponsiveness.[11] In another study of chronic schizophrenic patients, those who used marihuana had a lower rate of hospital admissions than those who used no drugs at all. They said cannabis helped them with anxiety, depression, and insomnia.[12] These contrary impressions may result from the differing effects of different cannabinoids. Whole smoked marihuana may be more comfortable to use than dronabinol (delta-9-THC), especially for schizophrenic patients, because cannabidiol neutralizes the capacity of delta-9-tetrahydrocannabinol to induce anxiety. Perhaps some schizophrenic patients find whole smoked marihuana useful because they are more sensitive to cannabidiol than to THC effects.[13]

11. V. Peralta and M. J. Cuesta, "Influence of Cannabis Abuse on Schizophrenic Psychopathology," *Acta Psychiatrica Scandinavica* 85:2 (February 1992): 127–130.

12. R. Warner, D. Taylor, J. Wright, et al., "Substance Use Among the Mentally Ill: Prevalence, Reasons for Use, and Effects on Illness," *American Journal of Orthopsychiatry* 64 (1994): 30–39.

13. Rats given the drug apomorphine develop stereotyped sniffing and biting behavior. Drugs with known antipsychotic activity in humans suppress this behavior; in

In a published clinical account, nineteen-year-old Ms. A was admitted to a psychiatric hospital because of aggressiveness, self-injury, incoherent thoughts, and auditory hallucinations:

During her first hospitalization at the age of seventeen years, she had been successfully treated with haloperidol (5 mg per day) but showed amenorrhea, galactorrhea, and weight gain after chronic treatment with the drug (2.5 to 7.5 mg/day) for eighteen months. The medication was tentatively stopped twice, but the symptoms returned. The second withdrawal trial led to the present hospitalization. At this time she was assessed by two psychiatrists who used the structured clinical interview for *DSM-III-R* [the standard diagnosis manual of the American Psychiatric Association]. Both agreed with the diagnosis of schizophrenia.

During the first four days of hospitalization, Ms. A received placebo plus usual environmental support measures. From days 4 to 30, she received cannabidiol dissolved in corn oil and packed inside gelatin capsules. The dose was progressively increased up to 1,500 mg/day in two divided doses. Cannabidiol intake was then replaced by placebo for four days. After that, haloperidol (5 mg/day) administration was started, and the dose was increased to 12.5 mg/day. Dose adjustments were determined by the clinical evaluation of the patient. During periods of great agitation and/or anxiety, diazepam 10 mg P.O. was administered. After one week of cannabidiol treatment, the mean daily dose of diazepam was reduced from 16.3 to 5.7 mg/day.

During the study, Ms. A was evaluated by two psychiatrists who used the Brief Psychiatric Rating Scale (BPRS) and the UKU

---

one experiment researchers found that cannabidiol also suppresses it. Another characteristic correlated with antipsychotic activity is a tendency to increased secretion of the hormone prolactin, which is also produced by cannabidiol. Some researchers have even suggested that cannabidiol belongs to the same group as the atypical antipsychotic drugs, including the highly effective clozapine. See A. W. Zuardi, J. A. Rodrigues, and J. M. Cunha, "Effects of Cannabidiol in Animal Models Predictive of Antipsychotic Activity," *Psychopharmacology* 104 (1991): 260–264.

Table 1   Raw Scores of BPRS and IOSPI and the Percentage of the Maximum
Score of BPRS Factors, Before and After Treatments

	BPRS		
Drug	Open	Blind	IOSPI
1st Placebo (Day 4)	42	50	16
Cannabidiol (Week 4)	13	20	5
2nd Placebo (Day 4)	17	30	10
Haloperidol (Week 4)	16	23	7

*Abbreviations: BPRS = Brief Psychiatric Rating Scale; IOSPI = Interactive
Observation Scale for Psychiatric Inpatients.

Reproduced from A. W. Zuardi, S. L. Morais, F. S. Guimarães, and R. Mechoulam, "Antipsychotic Effect of Cannabidiol," Letters to the Editor, *Journal of
Clinical Psychiatry* 56 (October 1995): 486.

Side Effect Rating Scale for psychoactive drugs. Interviews were
videotaped, and at the end of the study, the tapes were presented,
blindly and in a random sequence, to another psychiatrist, who
completed the BPRS. The patient was also evaluated independently by two nurse auxiliaries who used the Interactive Observation Scale for Psychiatric Inpatients (IOSPI) after daily observation periods of six hours.

The decrease in scores for the three measures after four weeks
of cannabidiol therapy was as follows: open BPRS, 69 percent;
blind BPRS, 60 percent; IOSPI, 69 percent. After cannabidiol
withdrawal, there was a trend toward worsening of the symptoms. The improvement obtained with cannabidiol was not increased by haloperidol treatment (decrease from baseline after
four weeks of haloperidol therapy: open BPRS, 62 percent; blind
BPRS, 54 percent; IOSPI, 56 percent). The improvement with
cannabidiol treatment was observed in all items of the BPRS, including those more closely related to psychotic symptoms, such
as "thought disturbance" and "hostility-suspiciousness," making

BPRS Factor (% of the Maximum Score)				
Thought Disturbance	Hostility-Suspiciousness	Anxiety-Depression	Activation	Anergia
62.5%	83.3%	62.5%	58.3%	31.3%
25.0%	33.3%	18.8%	16.7%	0.0%
31.3%	58.3%	12.5%	16.7%	6.3%
18.8%	41.7%	18.8%	25.0%	12.5%

it improbable that nonspecific anxiolytic action was responsible for the antipsychotic drug effect detected (table 1).

The finding that cannabidiol was well tolerated during this study confirms previous reports. A one-year follow-up showed a relapse associated with the reduction of haloperidol dose to 5 mg/day.[14]

Given the fact that 1 percent of the population suffers from schizophrenia and the serious limitations and side effects of existing antipsychotic drugs, the possibility that cannabidiol is an antipsychotic agent should be explored further.

SYSTEMIC SCLEROSIS (SCLERODERMA)

Scleroderma is an incurable disease of unknown origin in which various organs of the body are damaged by fibrosis—the replacement of normal tissue with scar or connective tissue. Often the first sign of the disease is Raynaud's phenomenon, a constriction of small blood vessels in the fingers and toes after exposure to cold, emotional stress, or tobacco smoke. Eventually fingers and hands become swollen and

14. A. W. Zuardi, S. L. Morais, F. S. Guimarães, and R. Mechoulam, "Antipsychotic Effect of Cannabidiol," Letters to the Editor, *Journal of Clinical Psychiatry* 56 (October 1995): 485–486.

the skin thickens, forming ugly patches on the face, hands, and feet. As the disease progresses, it affects the joints, causing arthritis-like pain and imprisoning the body in what Sir William Osler called "an ever-tightening cage of steel." In the most severe cases, scleroderma can threaten life by attacking the blood vessels, lungs, kidneys, and heart.

In many cases the internal organs most severely affected are those of the digestive system. Eating is often difficult because of puckering around the mouth and hardening and narrowing of the esophagus. More than half the patients develop such symptoms as severe heartburn, regurgitation of stomach contents, and difficulty in swallowing solid food. Other symptoms result from loss of muscle tone in the stomach and mobility in the small intestine.

Joe Hutchins is a fifty-one-year-old man who received the diagnosis of systemic sclerosis (scleroderma) thirty-two years ago. For the past twenty-one years he has been using marihuana to relieve the symptoms:

> My symptoms began in late 1963, while I was serving in the U.S. Navy in Charleston, South Carolina. After returning from a tour of duty aboard a minesweeper, I noticed that my hands were turning blue and discolored in the coolness of the morning. Within a few weeks some of my fingers became ulcerated, and I was admitted to a naval hospital. After months of diagnostic tests and skin biopsies, my doctor told me I had a disorder called Raynaud's phenomenon, in which blood vessels suddenly contract in the cold and cut off blood flow to the fingers and toes. He said I could live a normal life span but would have to stop smoking, because nicotine contracts the blood vessels. I gave up my two-pack-a-day cigarette habit and have never smoked tobacco since.
>
> I was given a medical discharge from the Navy and married in 1965. Despite the illness I had three healthy children between 1966 and 1971. I worked for a while as a millwright constructing power plants for electric utilities, but my hands became painful in the cold, so I trained as a machinist and went to work for

General Electric in Lynn, Massachusetts. Although I did not like working in a factory, at least it was warm there.

But eventually my hands became so swollen that they looked like little boxing gloves. The knuckles were numb, and I could not make a fist. I was finding it difficult to swallow solid food, because it became stuck in my lower esophagus. Every meal was pure hell. By November 1973 my weight had fallen to 150 pounds on a six-foot frame, and my esophagus was no longer function- ing. I was admitted to St. Elizabeth's Hospital in Boston, where a surgeon told me I had scleroderma—a disease of the connective tissue that is one of the causes of Raynaud's phenomenon. He said he could remove the esophagus and replace it with a seg- ment of my intestine, but there was no guarantee that this would work. The alternative was to insert a feeding tube directly into my stomach. Both prospects were horrifying.

Then friends who used marihuana told me it might improve my appetite and help me swallow. I had always refused mari- huana before, being a straight person who didn't think much of people who used illegal drugs. But this time I tried it as a last resort. The relief was dramatic. My appetite improved, and food didn't lodge in my esophagus so often. I no longer feared meals, and I gained twenty pounds. Marihuana also helped with other symptoms of scleroderma. Eventually I told my doctor, and he said I should continue if it allowed me to put off surgery. Now, when I can, I smoke several joints a day.

In 1978 I was hospitalized again, and my esophagus was di- lated with rubber tubes. Since then I have had this operation performed about once every two years. Together with marihuana, it allows me to eat fairly normally. But the procedure is risky— the esophagus can be perforated.

The same year my esophagus was first dilated, I left General Electric to live on total disability payments from the Veterans' Administration. My physical symptoms had become worse be- cause connective tissue was slowly being destroyed. My hands were constantly cold and blue and gradually becoming deformed.

My mouth puckered, and the oral opening became smaller and tighter. A dentist made a device that I would insert in my mouth to stretch it—a very uncomfortable procedure. I lost the hair on my lower legs and developed skin ulcerations that still persist. But the mental symptoms were worst, especially the nightmarish depression and the loss of the will or capacity for action.

During those years I took many drugs besides marihuana, including Vasodilan [isoxsuprine, a blood vessel dilator], Librium and Valium [chlordiazepoxide and diazepam, anti-anxiety drugs], Tofranil and Elavil [imipramine and amitriptyline, antidepressants]. I used Darvon [propoxyphene, an opioid] for the pain and swelling in my hands, Seconal [secobarbital] for insomnia, and Ritalin [methylphenidate, a stimulant] for daytime fatigue. At times I also took twelve to twenty-four aspirin a day, along with antacids and Tagamet [cimetidine, an ulcer treatment]. When I left General Electric I was taking seven different medications daily. Looking back on it, I can't imagine how I functioned at all. I was a legal junkie, addicted for many years.

In the spring of 1981 I was admitted to the psychiatric ward of a VA hospital and withdrawn from all the drugs. For three weeks I lay in bed and sweated uncontrollably, unable to focus or think. Before leaving I began biofeedback training, and through relaxation techniques and breathing exercises I managed to raise the temperature in my fingers from 75 to 80 degrees. But a month after discharge from the hospital I attempted suicide by ingesting several bottles of Valium, Darvon, and other drugs. I soon ended up in the VA hospital again, but left after ten days. Now I refuse to take any more prescribed drugs. I only want to use the one drug that helps me, marihuana.

After my last hospitalization I continued to smoke marihuana and began to feel better. My mouth opening widened, and the circulation in my fingers and toes improved. The temperature of my hands returned nearly to normal, and they did not become deformed any further. But the biggest improvement was in my mental health. I was less depressed and anxious and could work on my remaining depression and anxiety in psychotherapy.

Now I believe that some of the most serious symptoms of scleroderma can be managed more effectively with marihuana than with any conventional drug or combination of drugs. When I have to thrust my finger down my throat to regurgitate stuck food, I smoke marihuana and I can resume eating. Marihuana also relieves the nausea I feel after throwing up. It relaxes the smooth muscles surrounding my veins and arteries and allows better circulation of the blood. It also gives my mouth more elasticity and relieves mild to moderate pain, especially from swelling and stiffness of the joints. It relieves anxiety and depression without the horrifying side effects of other drugs.

In 1981 I began treatment with a psychologist who recommended that I try to obtain marihuana legally. The next year I began to ask the VA for legal marihuana. I have been repeatedly refused. I joined NORML [National Organization for the Reform of Marijuana Laws] and met many interesting people who favor the medical and personal use of marihuana and the reform of marihuana laws. I continued to smoke regularly, and in 1984 I was arrested on my own property for possession with intent to distribute (later revised to possession and manufacture).

The judge would not allow a defense of medical necessity, but I testified about my suicide attempt and the effects of marihuana. I was found guilty and remanded to the state mental hospital for fifteen days, then released and sentenced to a fine and probation. I appealed and received a new trial, but the judge again rejected the defense of medical necessity. The president of the Scleroderma Association testified about my disease, and my probation officer testified that I had been trying to obtain marihuana legally. I was found guilty of possession and manufacture of marihuana and sentenced to thirty days, followed by probation.

The state did everything it could to prevent my appeal from being heard — even denying the existence of documents that had already been presented as evidence at trial. Finally, in 1990, the Supreme Judicial Court of Massachusetts rejected my appeal by a vote of five to two. The dissent by the chief justice made me feel a little better, but I prepared myself for thirty days in jail.

My lawyer said that he and his firm would pursue a pardon from the governor. By this time I had moved to Washington State, where my doctor sponsored my request to receive marihuana through the federal government's Compassionate Investigational New Drug Program. Then a very uncompassionate President Bush axed the program. The *Boston Globe* published a moving editorial about my case under the title "Stone Cold Justice," and eventually I was pardoned. Partly because of the publicity about my situation, marihuana activists in Massachusetts succeeded in getting a therapeutic marihuana law passed. Unfortunately, the law will be ineffective until the federal government lifts its ban.

I have gained strength and life from a medicine put on this earth by God for all who are in need of it. He did not want us to be persecuted or condemned by society for the use of this wonderful plant. If I had to do it over again I would have started smoking marihuana in 1964. But now, my hope of procuring a legal prescription for smokable marihuana has become dimmer and dimmer. Until that day comes, I will remain stripped of the liberty, dignity, and peace of mind that are my rights as an American.

CROHN'S DISEASE

Crohn's disease is a rare but devastating chronic recurrent inflammation of the digestive tract, especially the small and large intestines. The intestinal wall becomes thickened and ulcerated in patches. Patients may develop abscesses (pockets of pus), fissures (cracks in the bowel wall), and fistulas (abnormal passages between parts of the intestine and between the intestine and the skin). The inside of the intestines may be narrowed so much that passage is obstructed. Common symptoms are cramps, nausea and vomiting, diarrhea, rectal bleeding, and loss of appetite and weight. Other parts of the body may also be affected, with symptoms that include skin disorders, eye inflammation, and arthritis.

Crohn's disease is treated mainly with the anti-inflammatory drugs mesalamine and sulfasalazine or with corticosteroids, which can be used for only a limited time. Most patients eventually need surgery to drain an abscess, free an obstruction, stop bleeding, or remove damaged parts of the intestine. Intravenous feeding may be necessary for weeks or even months at a time. Although symptoms fluctuate, the disease is chronic and usually responds less well to treatment as it progresses. The death rate is 5 to 10 percent.

Teresa Fasulo developed Crohn's disease when she was twenty-seven and soon discovered that marihuana, which she had been using recreationally, gave her symptomatic relief:

> When I started a new job recently, I realized the significance of my medical marihuana use. I had looked long and hard for the right work and career atmosphere, and I had found a place where I could excel in a variety of capacities. Unfortunately, on my first day I learned that the company required a drug screen before employment and yearly afterward. In a few hours I would have to urinate in a cup.
>
> I have no objection to drug screening in general; part of my job will be scheduling such tests, and certainly they are necessary for at least some employees, such as truck drivers. But it is absurd to include marihuana in the same screens as the addictive narcotics and cocaine. I feel entrapped and invaded and wonder what to do given marihuana's illegality. It has helped me like no other drug.
>
> My symptoms began in 1989: terrible diarrhea, cramping, nausea, and a feeling of fullness that deterred me from eating. The bowel incontinence was the most frightening part of it. Having "accidents" at the age of twenty-seven was not my idea of fun, nor was going to the bathroom thirty times a day. Not to mention being able to *feel* your intestines, from duodenum to colon. I saw a doctor who said I had colitis and prescribed Compazine [prochlorperazine] for the nausea. It only nauseated me even more and didn't relieve the "sloshing" feeling inside.
>
> By 1990, with a real job and medical insurance, I was able to consult a specialist, and in 1991 I was finally given the diagnosis of Crohn's disease. For a couple of years after that they were try-

ing out various drugs, but I was not medicated properly. When I moved to Boston in 1993 I was finally able to secure the help and medication I needed. Nevertheless, I ended up in a hospital with severe abdominal pain and inflammation and almost complete obstruction of the digestive tract. The disease had progressed to a point where the only option was intravenous feeding. It gave me complete relief, but I couldn't live a normal life that way.

For me the ultimate psychological challenge of this disease involves food. I was raised to adore food. My mother, my sister, and I can talk for hours about food and its preparation. Since my illness, it has been hard to develop an appetite at times for fear of what the food might do. During an inflammatory attack, I can eat only liquids and what is essentially mush. But I am determined not to have to give up the taste of food. Also, I have to be careful to eat regularly so as not to lose weight. Marihuana has been essential in helping me to eat normally and maintain my interest in food.

I discovered that marihuana helped almost as soon as the symptoms began. I developed a "joint before and after dinner" routine, and at first it was the only thing that kept me eating. Even a small amount of marihuana eliminated my post-dinner cramping entirely, relaxing me instantly. Now I take ten pills a day of mesalamine, an anti-inflammatory drug. I am also supposed to take Zantac [ranitidine] for the stomach upset and irritation, a cortisone enema foam, B¹² shots, and vitamin D. When the symptoms flare up for a long time, I have to take prednisone [a powerful corticosteroid]. This is the only drug that really seems to control the symptoms, but it has serious long-term side effects. All the other drugs have more side effects than marihuana, and they don't attack the disease itself but only relieve the symptoms. Whenever I can, I substitute a marihuana cigarette for Zantac. I believe that in the long run marihuana is less harmful. It has fewer side effects than all the other drugs and provides the best relief for my symptoms; it also helps me to maintain a perspective on the illness and on my life.

DIABETIC GASTROPARESIS

One long-term effect of diabetes, especially the kind that begins early in life (sometimes referred to as juvenile or Type I diabetes), is damage to nerve fibers of the autonomic nervous system. This system controls the gastrointestinal tract, among other things, and three-fourths of people with diabetes have gastrointestinal symptoms. One common syndrome is diabetic gastroparesis (the word means paralysis of the stomach), a disorder in which food remains in the stomach because of a failure of peristalsis, the natural contraction and relaxation of muscles that moves it along. The resulting symptoms include bloating, belching, nausea, vomiting, a sense of fullness, and appetite loss. Some serious consequences are malnourishment and loss of control over blood sugar levels. Patients are advised to avoid foods that slow gastric emptying and are given prescriptions for agents that speed it up, such as metoclopramide (Reglan) and cisapride (Propulsid). In the most severe cases surgery is attempted. None of the standard treatments works particularly well.

The following account is by a thirty-seven year old man who suffers from this syndrome:

In 1963, when I was five, I was diagnosed with diabetes mellitus after falling into a three-day coma. By the time I was hospitalized, my blood sugar was so high that all the veins in my body had collapsed. I have been dependent on insulin ever since, and it is a miracle that I am alive today to write this. My purpose is to inform other diabetics about a treatment for one particular diabetic complication.

I am one of those diabetics who is regarded as "brittle" because our blood sugar fluctuates wildly and almost uncontrollably. The resulting poor blood circulation and nerve damage (neuropathy) affect every part of the body, causing a myriad of symptoms. The one that concerns me here is the loss of function in the gut that occurs after many years of nerve and circulatory damage. The muscles of the GI tract, especially the stomach, are unable to move food through my system. It's called diabetic gastroparesis. The food sits in the stomach and causes bloating, acid buildup, and nausea, which may lead to vomiting. If this goes untreated, it can be life-threatening. Blood sugar quickly rises to dangerous levels, and the resulting dehydration almost always leads to hospitalization for as much as a week.

This condition must be fairly common since the pharmaceutical companies make two medications specifically designed to treat it, Reglan and Propulsid. Reglan is effective but very sedating. I used it for eight years, and I feel almost as though I slept through those years. It also caused me to lose equilibrium and contributed to a loss of sexual functioning. Propulsid, which I have been taking for about two years, does not have these side effects, but it doesn't move food through my system nearly as well, even at the double dose I am taking now. Another drawback is the cost of $160 a month, which is a real hardship for someone living on a fixed income.

I take my medication as prescribed, but in addition, when I can, I have begun to smoke a small amount of cannabis twenty minutes before each meal, usually just a couple of hits from a pipe. This outlawed drug makes the prescribed medication more effective. The bloating, the nausea, and the feeling of fullness go away, with practically no side effects. For the first time in years I can sit down to a meal and actually feel like eating (to see what I mean, try eating a full meal when you are already full from having just eaten).

The only problem I have with cannabis is that the supply is unreliable, and street prices are just ridiculous. Most of the time I cannot find it or cannot afford to pay the going rate. And I am made to feel like a criminal for seeking effective treatment for a potentially life-threatening condition. Someone who is dying from a chronic degenerative disease should not have to face incarceration because an effective medication for that disease has been made illegal by the government. I am only asking to be allowed to raise a small patch in my own yard for my own personal use. Who is harmed by that? Meanwhile, I hope I can help improve the quality of life for others suffering from gastroparesis by sharing my experience with cannabis.

PSEUDOTUMOR CEREBRI

Pseudotumor cerebri is an uncommon disorder characterized by abnormally high pressure of the cerebrospinal fluid (CSF) because the fluid is being produced at an accelerated rate or its outflow is being slowed. The underlying cause is unknown. The symptoms, which may include headaches, nausea, vomiting, and visual disturbances, resemble those of a brain tumor—thus the name. The patient's vision may be endangered by papilledema (swelling of the optic disk). The disorder is three times more common in women than in men, and it may last from several months to a lifetime.

None of the available treatments is especially effective, and the high rate of spontaneous recovery makes the evaluation of treatments difficult. Patients are sometimes given corticosteroids and high doses of diuretics to reduce fluid pressure. Frequent lumbar punctures (spinal taps) may be required to drain off CSF. In serious cases surgery is performed to insert a tube to shunt fluid from the brain into the abdominal cavity. As a last resort, when vision is seriously threatened and other treatments have failed, a surgeon may make an incision in the sheath of the optic nerve to relieve the pressure of papilledema.

Lori Horn is a twenty-nine-year-old woman with pseudotumor cerebri who has used marihuana recreationally since the age of eighteen. Here is her story:

> About four years ago I decided to quit using marihuana because the bills were becoming hard to pay. After five months of abstinence I began to develop severe headaches and disturbances in my vision (spots before my eyes). I went to see an optometrist, thinking I might need glasses. He sent me to a hospital ophthalmologist, who found acute pressure behind my eyes and three pinprick hemorrhages. I was rushed to an emergency

room, where a neurologist said I might have a brain tumor. Fortunately, X-rays, CAT scans, blood tests, and a spinal tap all came back negative. At that point I was given the diagnosis of pseudotumor cerebri. The doctors prescribed Motrin [ibuprofen, a nonsteroidal anti-inflammatory drug], prednisone [a powerful steroid], and Diamox [acetazolamide, a diuretic].

The prednisone made me extremely moody; my face swelled up and I gained an enormous amount of weight. The Diamox caused muscle cramps and made my leaky bladder worse. Motrin did almost nothing for my headaches. I was told I might need surgery (which didn't always work) to prevent blindness. I began to live in fear of losing my sight; I had nightmares and cried for hours.

By now it had been eight months since I'd last used marihuana, so I decided to smoke a joint. It was almost magical. For the next two weeks I had no headaches, no disturbances in vision. Doctors even said my eyes looked better (the papilledema had disappeared). When I told my neurologist, he didn't seem very interested but said, "If it works, use it."

Against doctors' orders, I quit taking all the prescribed medications and began smoking a joint once every few days instead. Now I find that I get headaches and visual disturbances if I go more than a week without a good joint. The more potent the marihuana, the longer my eyes remain healthy. They look so good now that all talk of shunt surgery and spinal taps to relieve pressure has ended.

My family has watched the miracle of my marihuana use, and they know it helps me. I thank God it was there as an alternative to the knife and to drugs like prednisone. I only wish I had a doctor to back me up, but the hospital where I was treated offered me no support, not even written documentation of my self-medication and its miraculous effects. When I heard about you I decided to tell you my story. It touches my heart to find that there really are people who care about people like me. What

can I do, where can I go? I've been charged with possession once
already. I pray it doesn't happen again.

TINNITUS

Tinnitus is a ringing, whistling, hissing, or buzzing sound in the
ear with no external source. The auditory nerve is apparently responding to a stimulus that comes from inside the head or within the ear
itself. It is a symptom of many ear disorders but also occurs without
a known cause. The noise can sometimes be drowned out by masking it with a radio, television, headphones, or other device. After the
masking agent is removed, tinnitus may remain quiescent for a while
because of a process known as neural inhibition. Unfortunately, masking is often ineffective, and there is no cure for tinnitus of unknown
origin.

Greg Gindlesperger is a thirty-nine-year-old man who was born
with total deafness in his left ear, a 50-percent reduction of hearing
in his right ear, and severe tinnitus:

> When I was in third grade, teachers were alarmed by my inability
> to learn. My parents took me to my family doctor, who thought
> I was hyperactive and put me on Ritalin [methylphenidate]. It
> wasn't until later that they found out I was deaf in my left ear and
> had limited hearing in my right ear. I would get severe headaches,
> but the worst part was the ringing in my ears. Sometimes it com-
> pletely dominated my thoughts. The frustration of not being able
> to hear above the ringing causes irrational behavior and brings
> on severe head pain. It makes me feel that if I can't stop the ring-
> ing, my head will blow up. When I was a child it was so severe
> at times that I would lie in bed and cry.
>
> I was fitted with a hearing aid to amplify other sounds so that
> the ringing would not dominate everything—like turning up the
> TV to drown out the radio. But often I just could not tune it out.
> Faced with a loss of jobs and friends, I looked for people who

could accept me and found them in the rock-and-roll crowd. They liked loud music, and loud was fine with me. No one could hear well with the music so loud, so I fit right in. This group smoked pot, too, and that is how I came to learn about it. At first I had no idea pot could help me, because I smoked only at parties and concerts, where the loud music dominated everything. Soon I was married with a child on the way and went to work at General Electric, where drug testing would be done. Obviously pot smoking was out.

My wife and I had a baby and a new house. In most families this is a time of joy, but for me it was almost pure hell. Babies make lots of noise, and crying, for some reason, gives me severe headaches. Can you imagine hoping that you will go completely deaf so that your child's crying won't drive you to suicide? I became depressed and had no interest in the outside world. I felt I was beginning to lose my sanity. I felt so bad for my family that for a while leaving was the only way I could think of to save them from the embarrassment of having to deal with me. I went off to California, but I called home daily to combat the loneliness, and I soon returned.

After my return an old friend stopped over, said I needed to mellow out, and invited me to smoke pot with him. I hadn't smoked since my marriage, and I thought we were a little old to still be getting high, but I decided to go along. To my surprise, my headache and the ringing in my ears slowly faded away, and I was able to hear normal sounds. It still works. When I smoke marihuana, the ringing and pain go away almost immediately, the background noise diminishes, and I can hear what I am trying to listen to. It's as though an improperly tuned station is now tuned right and the music is coming through clearly. I have been smoking marihuana for so long now that I feel no euphoria — just the loss of the ringing and headaches.

Unfortunately, marihuana is expensive. The only way to have my medicine and not go broke was to grow my own. I built a four-by-four room in the basement hidden behind a closet and grew marihuana there. Life was good until one Saturday afternoon when the police came and served a search warrant. They said that someone had told them I was growing pot, and they used a heat-seeking device to corroborate the story. I was charged with possession and manufacture of marihuana, a felony. I have been in and out of court for two years and now face a three- to five-year sentence. Meanwhile I am unable to use the medicine that helps me most.[15]

Marihuana is rarely mentioned in the research literature on tinnitus, except to suggest that it can precipitate or aggravate the disorder. However, one text notes that "at least one patient" found marihuana to be the only drug that relieved her symptoms.[16]

VIOLENCE

Our understanding of the relationship between marihuana use and violence has come full circle over the past sixty years. During the 1930s Harry Anslinger, the first director of the Federal Bureau of Narcotics (predecessor of the Drug Enforcement Administration), vigorously promoted the view that cannabis use led to all sorts of mayhem. The plot of the film *Reefer Madness*, perhaps the best-known product of the government-backed marihuana "educational" campaign of the 1930s, depended on marihuana's supposed capacity to induce violence and sexual debauchery. Even as the film was being produced, the Army conducted a study of soldiers in the Panama Canal Zone which demonstrated that marihuana did not cause violence or present a threat to military discipline. The Army's report advised against "recommendations . . . to prevent the sale or use of marihuana."[17] A few years later, researchers in India pointed out that "so far as premedi-

15. Since this account was written, Gindlesperger has been sentenced to three years in a state prison and ordered to pay a fine of $15,000.
16. *Tinnitus: Pathology and Management,* ed. M. Kitahara (Tokyo and New York: Igaku-shoin, 1988), 65.
17. J. F. Siler et al., "Marijuana Smoking in Panama," *Military Surgery* 73 (1933): 279–280.

tated crime is concerned, especially that of a violent nature, hemp drugs . . . may not only not lead to it, but actually act as deterrence. . . . One of the important actions of these drugs is to quieten and stupefy the individual so there is no tendency to violence. . . . The result of continued . . . use of these drugs in our opinion is to make the individual timid rather than lead him to commit a crime of a violent nature." [18]

Although no one makes the claim today that cannabis causes violence, its capacity to inhibit violent behavior is often disregarded. Our first direct experience of this occurred several years ago in Kuala Lumpur, Malaysia, where one of us (L.G.) was examining a prisoner in Pudu Prison. He was an American teacher in his late thirties who faced the death penalty for possession of marihuana, which he used to treat a severe chronic spastic condition that resulted from a mountain-climbing accident. More than a hundred people had already been hanged for drug offenses in Malaysia, and he would have been the first American.[19] When asked how he managed without cannabis in prison, he replied that Pudu Prison was "the easiest place in the world to get marihuana." Guards sold it to prisoners, not only to earn money, but to prevent prison disturbances. We have since become aware that many prison officials in the United States share the view that prisoners who use cannabis are less likely to be troublemakers.

The value of this property is suggested by the following account from a man who probably suffers from what the American Psychiatric Association's diagnostic manuals have called Intermittent Aggressive Disorder (*DSM-III*) or Organic Personality Disorder, Aggressive Type (*DSM-IV*):

My name is Collin Bosiger, I'm thirty-six years old, and I suffer from acute rage syndrome. Ever since I can remember, I've

18. R. N. Chopra and G. S. Chopra, "The Present Position of Hemp Drug Addiction in India," *Indian Medical Research Memoirs* 31 (1939): 92.

19. For a more detailed account of this trial, see L. Grinspoon, "A Brief Account of My Participation as a Witness in the Trial of Kerry Wiley," *International Journal on Drug Policy* 2:5 (March–April 1991): 11–12.

had trouble controlling violent emotions and behavior. Since my mother was an abusive alcoholic, my sister and I were adopted when I was three. Always in trouble, I spent most of my adolescence in a variety of juvenile facilities, including Virginia's largest and best known reform school and penitentiary. In one place, where they were experimenting with behavior modification, they had me make and wear a sign that said in huge bright letters: "I am an atomic bomb. Watch out, I may explode on you." I have found that marihuana keeps me from being that atomic bomb.

I was exposed to marihuana at an early age but wasn't able to adopt it as a habit until I was out on my own at twenty-three. I began to buy small amounts whenever I could. By my late twenties it occurred to me that I hadn't been in as much trouble as before. My life was actually going well. I had a job, money, new things—it was great. I still had strong emotions, but I was able to control them and not blow up. I have come to realize that the difference very much depends on marihuana.

Here is the kind of thing that happens all the time. Once a friend and I were having difficulty putting a transmission in a car, something I do often as an auto mechanic. I was getting so frustrated and angry that my helper backed off and said it was too dangerous to stay under that car with me. He suggested that I have a bit of herb. I came back afterward and the transmission slipped right in. We were bolting it within a few minutes.

When marihuana becomes unavailable I feel anxious all the time. My muscles tense up and my eyes seem about to bulge out of my head. During one of these dry spells I got so angry I started hitting the walls of my house with my fist until I'd completely destroyed several walls and broken my hand in the process. At least that time I didn't hurt my wife. During another dry spell, in April 1989, she wasn't so lucky; I hit her and was arrested. The next week I was hauled in again for assault on two other people.

The court forced me to get professional help. My psychiatrists diagnosed me with a variant of Tourette's syndrome and put me on Zoloft [sertraline], Prozac [fluoxetine], and Ritalin [methylphenidate]. None of it helped. Next I was sent to a neurologist who said I had adult attention deficit disorder. He gave me more Ritalin, plus Haldol [haloperidol].

But the doctors' drugs never did work. All that stuff is a waste. Marihuana is what works, but when I explain that I get a lot of resistance. If my doctors could walk a mile in my shoes, they would authorize my use of it.

POST-TRAUMATIC STRESS DISORDER

Post-traumatic stress disorder (PTSD) results from an overwhelming assault on the mind and emotions involving a threat of death or serious injury or damage to one's physical integrity. The cause may be a natural disaster, an accident, or a human action. There are three kinds of symptoms. First, victims are often edgy, irritable, easily startled, and constantly on guard—a group of symptoms often described as hyperarousal. The second set of symptoms is called intrusion. Victims involuntarily re-experience the traumatic event in the form of memories, nightmares, and flashbacks, during which they may feel or even act as though the event were recurring. They also suffer when they are exposed to anything that resembles, recalls, or symbolizes some aspect of the trauma. A third set of symptoms is emotional constriction or numbing—a need to avoid feelings and thoughts reminiscent of the trauma, a loss of normal emotional responses, or both. This emotional numbing often causes demoralization and isolation.

A Gulf War veteran describes his use of marihuana to treat PTSD complicated by a variety of other symptoms that have been labeled Desert Storm or Gulf War syndrome:

> I am a twenty-six-year-old Desert Storm veteran with a diagnosis of PTSD after combat exposure and a knee injury in the Persian Gulf theater. I was diagnosed in November 1991 by a Veterans' Administration physician after a series of job failures and personal difficulties.
>
> Many of my symptoms appeared soon after I returned. I had

nightmares, cold sweats, and panic attacks. I would instantly hit the ground when loud sounds went off in my direction, and there were terror episodes when I thought I smelled burning oil. There were also days on end when I could barely get out of bed, even to go to the bathroom.

I also had rashes on my feet, and the skin on my genitals started to crack and bleed. I lost my sense of smell and most of my sense of taste, so I neglected eating. I was put through a series of tests and diagnosed with Desert Storm syndrome. It seems we were exposed to a multitude of contaminants including nuclear, bio, depleted uranium, and some the Department of Defense is withholding from disclosure. Any combination of these might have been the cause of my symptoms, plus the shots we took to protect us from diseases and the nerve gas antidote (NAPT pills) given to front-line servicemen.

The doctor told me I had to start eating to build up my depleted immune system. I asked him how he expected me to do that, and he suggested I try cannabis to see if it gave me the munchies. I smoked about a quarter of a gram of high grade cannabis about a half hour before my next meal, and to my surprise I ate a full meal for the first time in nine months. The doctor documented this for my files.

As my therapy progressed, I started to gain self-confidence and come out from behind my shield. My night terrors and panic attacks became less frequent, and so did my fatigue, because I was eating better. Through my conversations with the counselors at the VA, I began to come to terms with what I did in combat. The doctors wanted to put me on Prozac to elevate my mood, but I refused. I told them that cannabis elevated my mood when I felt depressed or alone.

I was put into a National Guard unit to finish out my service time, and during a weekend drill I was given a random urinalysis that showed I was positive for THC. I was discharged dishonorably, and my military career was wrecked.

In 1992 I moved to California to start a new life, but I couldn't find a job. I went to the VA clinic in Oakland to register with a Gulf War registry. I told the physicians there that I smoked the equivalent of two joints a day to stimulate my appetite and get me through the day without panic attacks. When I did get a panic attack, I found that a quarter of a gram of high-grade marihuana made it subside in a few minutes; it was the same for sleeplessness due to nightmares. Shortly after that, I joined the Cannabis Action Network in Berkeley as a volunteer. I was given all the information on medical marihuana I needed to present to my doctors. I acted as a consultant to other cannabis patients, and through talking with them I helped to heal them and myself.

I am now employed full-time as a sales manager for one the most successful hemp companies in the United States. I am soon to be married. I still smoke marihuana for appetite stimulation. Cannabis has changed my life for the better. It has allowed me to deal with my situation and make the best of my limitations both physically and spiritually, without regrets or addiction.

PHANTOM LIMB PAIN

Almost everyone who has had a limb amputated experiences sensations that are interpreted by the brain as though they came from the missing (phantom) limb. In two-thirds of the cases these sensations include persistent pain, usually of a cutting, stabbing, or pricking nature. Phantom limb pain is treated, often inadequately, with the standard array of analgesics.

Richard E. Musty, professor of psychology at the University of Vermont, describes a graduate student's use of marihuana for the purpose:

> Deborah Finnegan-Ling, a doctoral student in the department of psychology at the University of Vermont, suffered a severe injury to her ankle while working with her husband on the family farm and eventually had to have her foot amputated. After the amputation she had classical phantom limb symptoms. She felt

as though the foot was still intact and she could wiggle her toes. She also had chronic dull pain punctuated by frequent attacks of sharp, stabbing, acute pain in the phantom foot. These attacks occurred without warning many times a day, often while she was lecturing, and forced her to stop whatever she was doing until the pain subsided. The attacks also woke her five or six times a night for a year after her surgery.

Deborah tried various treatments, including hypnosis and stimulation of the stump by warm water. She also tried a dozen different drugs, including anti-inflammatories, antidepressants, anticonvulsants, benzodiazepines, and opioid narcotics. All of them were either ineffective or had intolerable side effects. In the spring of 1993 I read *Marihuana, the Forbidden Medicine* [first edition] and suggested to Deborah that marihuana might help. She had smoked it when she was younger but felt that as a thirty-six-year-old mother of teenage daughters she could no longer do so. I suggested she ask her neurologist to prescribe Marinol. Much to my surprise, she returned with a prescription the next day.

I helped her work out a dosing regimen, since I was familiar with the literature on Marinol for cancer chemotherapy and had conducted marihuana smoking studies in my lab. She began by taking 5 mg one hour before dinner, 10 mg one hour before bedtime, and 5 mg on arising at 5 A.M. After two months she changed the dose to 10 mg one hour before bedtime and 10 mg on arising. Her ability to fall asleep improved almost immediately, and she slept a full night for the first time in over a year. The chronic dull pain decreased, and the number of acute pain attacks fell to less than one a day; sometimes she would go three or four days without one. Her appetite improved, and she gained three pounds in a few months.

Deborah has read most of the literature on phantom limb pain and decided to write a doctoral dissertation on the subject under my supervision. Together we prepared a study of her case and presented it in the summer of 1994 at a meeting of the International Cannabis Research Society, where it attracted a great deal of attention. After three years she is still using Marinol. It is still effective, and she has not developed tolerance.

ALCOHOLISM AND OTHER ADDICTIONS

Three to 10 percent of Americans will at some time in their lives be alcohol abusers. The medical and social costs run to tens of billions of dollars a year, more than the cost of cancer and respiratory disease combined. Alcoholism is not only the world's most common drug problem but one of the hardest to treat. The best approach is uncertain at every stage from diagnosis to precarious recovery. No two cases respond to the same handling.

Most drugs are not very useful, and some create a serious danger of dependence. A few alcoholics suffering from severe depression will be helped by antidepressants, but more often the depression results from alcohol abuse and clears up after withdrawal. The only drug now commonly given to recovering alcoholics is disulfiram (Antabuse), which prevents the body from breaking down and excreting alcohol normally. Acetaldehyde, a toxic metabolite, accumulates and causes nausea whenever the patient drinks. Disulfiram is useful only to alcoholics who are willing to keep taking it, and many are not. It is a treatment—or rather an aid to treatment—that will not work unless the patient is committed to long-term change and needs protection only against momentary lapses. Furthermore, great care is necessary in using disulfiram, as alcohol can be lethal to someone who is taking it.

It has been known since the nineteenth century that cannabis is useful to some alcoholics. In 1881 H. H. Kane noted that one of his patients, a thirty-eight-year-old Englishwoman, had taken up the use of hashish in a successful effort to replace alcohol, to which she had become addicted. She smoked hashish daily in a pipe and often said that if she wished she could stop using it without difficulty.[20] Although Kane's description of her physical condition does not suggest robust health, it must be kept in mind that she had been an alcoholic for

20. H. H. Kane, *Drugs That Enslave* (Philadelphia, 1881), 208–210.

some years before exchanging alcohol for cannabis. Dr. Kane thought she would have fared better if she had made the exchange earlier.

Perhaps some people need a consciousness-altering substance but can substitute cannabis for more dangerous drugs, with a resulting improvement in health. That seems to be true of Alan McLemore, whose story follows:

> I was a lawyer, and a good one. So good that I was variously known as "The Kid" or "The Eagle." Now I'm a federal prisoner, #05204-078, serving a six-and-a-half-year sentence for growing marihuana.
>
> I was born in April 1951 to a solidly middle-class WASP family. As the genetic cards go, I was dealt a pretty good hand, including (for what it's worth) an IQ that has consistently tested in the 150 range. But there was a joker in the deck—a condition described, inadequately, as depression. It has manifested itself in many ways, but most devastatingly as the disease of alcoholism.
>
> As far back as I can recall, I was moody and withdrawn. As a child I remember feelings of hopelessness, loneliness, anxiety, and impending doom. Sensations have always seemed too harsh: colors too bright, sounds too loud, odors too strong. I hated to get out of bed, even though I usually didn't sleep restfully. I rarely felt like doing anything and was often called lazy. I was also taken to a psychiatrist at the age of nine because of severe appetite problems. I preferred to stay as far away as possible from other kids and their play, which I found to be unbearably loud and raucous. All I wanted to do was read, which I did voraciously from an early age. School was an ordeal I dreaded. I often missed classes but usually managed to get straight A's anyway. At puberty I felt compelled to socialize more but still perceived myself as a clumsy outsider to an extent that went beyond normal adolescent angst.
>
> Then, at eighteen, I discovered beer. All of a sudden I felt *good*. People and things were transformed from tedious to fascinating. For the first time in my life I *wanted* to be around people, to do new and different things. In my first year of college, 1969,

I became actively interested in social issues, especially race and Vietnam. I picked up the guitar and began to play in rock and soul bands. In other words, I began to have a reasonably normal social life for the era, except that I seemed to drink a lot more than others did.

Toward the end of my freshman year in college my career as an alcoholic took a brief detour when I began to smoke marihuana. Like alcohol, marihuana made me feel good. Unlike alcohol, it gave me no hangovers and allowed me to make it to classes and tests on time. But it was hard to get and the quality was uneven. It was also *very* illegal: possession of even a single seed was a felony in my home state of Texas. Then I heard of "new scientific studies" purporting to show that marihuana was dangerous to the mind and body. (It wasn't until two decades later that I discovered that the "studies" were lies.) So, making the greatest mistake of my life, I chose alcohol over marihuana at age twenty-one. I was already vaguely aware that I had a problem, so I also made the first of many promises to myself that I would begin to limit my drinking.

Instead, I became a weekend binger. I knew that my behavior and drinking were often out of control, but I convinced myself that I was not an alcoholic because I could go for long periods between drinking bouts. I began law school in Austin in late 1973 and graduated with a gentleman's C average in 1977. During those years I was married for the first time and worked as a legal assistant to my hometown state representative (essentially a patronage job). I also began to drink more and more heavily. In late 1974 I was arrested for the first time for driving while intoxicated (DWI).

It was the evening of my younger brother's first wedding. At the reception I got drunk on champagne, and later I drove a friend into town to continue drinking. I was stopped for speeding, arrested, and taken to jail, loudly proclaiming my opinion of the officer and the police in general. I learned firsthand that the police don't always play by the rules, because when I refused to quiet down I was taken into a narrow cell by myself, shown a length of water hose, and again ordered to shut up. I obeyed orders and was released on bond after spending several hours in a cell with a gentleman who was trying to persuade me to have sex with him.

I got six months' probation and after that quit drinking for two whole months. But soon I began to drink more heavily than ever. In August 1977, when I moved back to my hometown to take a job as assistant district attorney, I had begun to drink heavily nearly every day. But I was good in the courtroom and was getting a reputation as a rising star. By the time I left the DA's office in August 1980, everyone thought I was headed for fame and fortune.

And so it seemed for a while. My practice and my income grew rapidly. Unfortunately, so did my drinking problem. I began to spend more and more time in the honky-tonks, the little run-down country and western bars east Texas is so full of. I kept a keg of beer on tap on my patio, and every evening after work I'd "relax" until I was ready to collapse into bed drunk. By late 1982 the signs were so obvious that even I couldn't ignore them. One morning, as I drank beer to calm my shakes, I admitted to myself that I had a problem. I saw my family doctor and told him I wanted to "moderate" my drinking. He recommended AA, and I attended many meetings, but it ultimately proved worthless to me. The simple fact was that without alcohol I *hurt*. I was miserable, back in the "normal" state I had known since birth.

I was spending more and more nights away from home and less and less time at the office. I had money problems and needed to borrow more and more heavily. By 1984 I knew I was in real trouble and saw a psychiatrist. He explained that my alcoholism was an attempt to self-medicate underlying depression. After hospitalizing me to dry out, he began to treat me with the antidepressants then available.

But nothing helped for long. My economic circumstances began to deteriorate, along with my reputation and legal abilities. My office building was repossessed, my first wife left me after ten years of marriage, and I was hospitalized several times for alcohol-related stomach problems. There were also more arrests for DWI, and in 1987 I was given a year on probation, during which I continued to drink, in violation of the court's order and common sense.

In 1988 I married a woman who was a cocaine addict, imagining that we could help each other. The marriage ended after two weeks when I got drunk and she ran off with her cocaine dealer. Shortly afterward I moved to my mother's place and again tried and failed to kick the alcohol habit.

In 1989 I married again, resumed my law practice, and bought a house. I also began to drink heavily again, and this time my life went to hell in months rather than years. From a few beers a night, I progressed to straight 190-proof Everclear in less than three months. I was arrested again while driving drunk, and during the scuffle I bruised a cop on the arm. I was charged with aggravated assault on a police officer and eventually got three years' probation.

Incredibly, I continued to drink. The house was repossessed, and my wife left me. I ended up living in a dilapidated trailer, drinking a quart of 101-proof whiskey a day, broke and sick. By August 1990 I had lived there for three months without paying rent. I often thought of suicide.

Then I met a guy who had access to street marihuana. Looking for a new way to oblivion, I started to smoke it and miraculously found that my craving for alcohol began to recede. I could wait until later and later in the day before starting to drink. By mid-September 1990 I had stopped drinking altogether, without pain or suffering or a trace of craving for alcohol—and also without headaches, mood swings, anxiety, sleep disturbances, and other symptoms of depression.

In 1992 I lost contact with my marihuana suppliers and relapsed badly into drinking for two months. At that time I got a prescription for Marinol, but my doctor wouldn't give me enough to quell my symptoms; he would only prescribe one ten-milligram pill per month. So I began to grow marihuana for myself. I supplied the location and the equipment, while a couple of friends supplied the seeds and the labor. I got what I needed to smoke, and they paid me enough to compensate for my expenses.

With the help of marihuana I put my life back together. I never drank again. By 1995 I owned a nice homestead which I had completely paid for, as well as several trucks, a race horse, and other toys too numerous to mention. My income had risen to $100,000 a year. My health was good. Life was great. I was active; I tended to my law practice and found what it was like to live a "normal" life. What a difference an herb makes.

All that came to an end on February 8, 1995, when I was arrested for "conspiracy to manufacture marihuana" in a military-style assault by soldiers with machine guns and helicopters. I was taken to jail, where my condition began to deteriorate, and I declared a hunger strike to protest the inhumanity of the drug war (I didn't tell the authorities that without THC it was difficult for me to eat). After I lost over thirty pounds, the federal magistrate signed an order for forced feeding, and the staff psychiatrist at the county jail prescribed 10 mg of Marinol daily. The Marinol worked: I regained appetite and weight, and the other symptoms of depression largely disappeared. I was forced to plead guilty to a felony; all my property was forfeited, and I lost my law license. But throughout the ordeal I remained mentally stable and physically healthy. I even found the woman of my dreams, a local community activist who visits me in jail to offer her support. We fell in love and are to be married.

Some people who are not alcoholic have learned to exchange the "social" use of alcohol for cannabis because they enjoy it more or believe that marihuana is safer and less addictive. But simple substitution probably does not explain cannabis use by people who have been addicted to alcohol. For one thing, alcohol intoxication is quite different from cannabis intoxication, and people who are comfortable with (and comforted by) the former do not necessarily enjoy the latter. McLemore's account suggests two other possibilities. He believes that he was using alcohol largely as a home remedy for depression. Alcohol use itself can cause depression, and a vicious spiral often develops—more depression, heavier drinking, deeper depression. As we have pointed out, cannabis can be used as a treatment for depression.

The other possibility is that, as McLemore also suggests, cannabis diminishes the craving for alcohol. Chuck Cass, whose story follows, believes it is useful for that reason.

> I am forty-four years old. I have a degree in computer science and am licensed as a high-pressure boiler operator, but I am currently unemployed and spend most of my time caring for my infant son.
>
> My drinking began at about the age of eleven. I came from a heavy drinking family and community, and it was easy to steal a few beers here and there for myself while the family was partying. Soon I tried my hand at brewing and succeeded in producing dandelion wine and a tasty banana brandy. By age fourteen I had found a sympathetic aunt who bought me pints of vodka. I spent most of my weekends riding my trailbike or snow machine with a pint of vodka tucked in my belt. By the next year my life as an alcoholic was well underway. My parents' marriage was breaking up, and I found great comfort in getting drunk with friends at weekend parties. We lived in a town on the Canadian border, and I found I could buy beer at many Canadian stores and drink at most bars there.
>
> By the time I was seventeen I would go with a buddy to a remote picnic area many Saturday afternoons and sit there until early evening, drinking half of a fifth of liquor each. Then we would get into my car and drive off to a dance or party for the night.
>
> My alcoholism continued through two marriages, although I was able to confine my drinking to weekends and holidays, and my job in the computer field never suffered.
>
> When I was in my early thirties my roadside-picnic buddy died of massive internal-organ problems; he had been drinking heavily nearly every day. This made me begin to think, and I realized I had a problem, too. I was drinking a half-gallon of rum during an evening of cards with friends, and my hangovers lasted three to

four days. This was when I discovered that smoking marihuana the morning after helped relieve the nausea and shakes. Soon I began to drink less and smoke more.

In my late thirties I made my first serious attempt to quit drinking. I began to smoke marihuana several times a day to neutralize the craving for alcohol. I knew that alcohol had many ill effects and marihuana had none. It was much easier to maintain a job and a home life while smoking.

Just before turning forty-two I allowed myself one more binge with alcohol, but for the past two years I have been smoking marihuana whenever I feel stressed out and in need of a drink. I feel much better physically, and I have no hangovers. I have cut down my smoking to two or three times a week. Recently I went two weeks without smoking at all, but near the end of this period my thoughts began to return to alcohol. I still need marihuana to keep those thoughts away.

We realize that anecdotal evidence can lead to false understandings. We have found only two people who would share their stories of using cannabis to free themselves of alcohol addiction. But they, as well as others addicted to opiates or tobacco, believe that cannabis can reduce craving. We have no idea how common or how powerful this capacity is, but further exploration would be worthwhile even if only a few highly motivated alcoholics and other addicts could benefit. After all, almost anyone who is sophisticated about both alcoholism and cannabis use would gladly exchange alcohol for marihuana.

The same can be said of other addictive drugs. The American physician J. B. Mattison, whom we have already mentioned as an early advocate of medical cannabis, asserted that in his practice it had "proved an efficient substitute for the poppy." One of his cases was "a naval surgeon, nine years a ten-grains-daily subcutaneous morphine taker . . . [who] recovered with less than a dozen doses" of a *Cannabis indica* preparation.[21] This use had already been reported two years

21. J. B. Mattison, "*Cannabis indica* as an Anodyne and Hypnotic," *St. Louis Medical Surgical Journal* 61 (1891): 266.

earlier by E. A. Birch, M.D., who treated a chloral hydrate addict and an opium addict with *Cannabis indica* in an experiment approaching modern research techniques. He replaced the drug of addiction with unidentified pills containing cannabis, which he then gradually withdrew. In each case Birch noted a prompt response with the return of appetite and sound sleep.[22]

S. Allentuck and K. M. Bowman, two psychiatrists who studied cannabis for the LaGuardia Commission, found in a study of forty-nine cases that when cannabis was substituted for opiates, "the withdrawal symptoms were ameliorated or eliminated sooner, the patient was in a better frame of mind, his spirits were elevated, his physical condition was more rapidly rehabilitated, and he expressed a wish to resume his occupation sooner."[23] About ten years later another pair of investigators, L. J. Thompson and R. C. Proctor, reported favorable results when they used pyrahexyl, a synthetic cannabis preparation, in the treatment of patients withdrawing from alcohol, barbiturates, and various narcotics. They agreed with Allentuck and Bowman that cannabis did not cause physiological dependence or withdrawal symptoms of its own.[24]

It is remarkable how little follow-up there has been on this suggestive early research. Large comprehensive clinical trials are clearly needed, but the prospects for such studies are poor. In addition to the general legal and institutional impediments to clinical marihuana research, there is a special obstacle in this case: many still wrongly regard marihuana itself as an addictive drug. That may explain the problems of Bill Young, a thirty-nine-year-old opiate addict, who tells his story here:

> I've now survived more than twenty years of heroin and opiate addiction. I've also withdrawn from opiates many times in many ways over the years, but I can never stay off for long. I guess I

22. E. A. Birch, "The Use of Indian Hemp in the Treatment of Chronic Chloral and Chronic Opium Poisoning," *Lancet* 1 (1889): 625.

23. S. Allentuck and K. M. Bowman, "The Psychiatric Aspects of Marihuana Intoxication," *American Journal of Psychiatry* 99 (1942): 250.

24. L. J. Thompson and R. C. Proctor, "Pyrahexyl in the Treatment of Alcoholic and Drug Withdrawal Conditions," *North Carolina Medical Journal*, 14 (1953): 520–523.

passed some point of no return long ago. The chronic and terrible pain of migraine headaches and a bad back led to my addiction, first to prescription pain pills such as Demerol [meperidine] and Dilaudid [hydromorphone], and then to heroin. The pain persists and sabotages every effort to stop.

For years many wise people begged me to try long-term methadone maintenance, and it turned out to be the best thing I've ever done. Although methadone didn't cure my addiction or eliminate the pain, it did change my life by getting me through each day with one safe, legal, long-lasting oral dose. The resulting stability has allowed my girlfriend and me to begin building a life together. The methadone program is private, and I pay for it myself, but political tampering here in Memphis now threatens to reverse my gains, redefine my success as failure, and send me back to my disease as a hopeless case.

I'm in danger of being kicked out, but not because the program is no longer working for me or because my doctors and counselors think it's a good idea to take me off methadone. The reason my good life may slip through my fingers is that those who would save the world from marihuana have found a new target for their crusade: registered addicts in methadone programs, who must, for sensible reasons, provide regular urine drug screens. Those screens were never meant to force anyone to leave treatment, but all that has changed, and I wouldn't take any sizable bets on my future.

It doesn't matter to the bureaucrats and police who are pressing for this crackdown that I've always been honest with the clinic about my medicinal marihuana use. From my first day of treatment, I told my doctors and counselors I believed nothing else worked as well to ease my two main sources of physical pain and aid my fight to keep from shooting up heroin and other opiates. Marihuana is not part of my problem but a big part of the solution. Of course, I can't obtain a prescription for marihuana, so by definition I am guilty of illicit drug use. Should that disqualify me from a treatment that has worked so well all these years?

Only opiates like methadone can really stop withdrawal symptoms (by blocking the shrieking opiate receptors in the addicted brain), but smoking very small amounts of marihuana does seem to calm my opiate craving. The mild change in consciousness produced by marihuana quiets the siren song of heroin. Beyond that, one small joint subdues the stabbing pain of my spasming lower back, which has been damaged by an arthritis-like disease. Sometimes it also aborts an oncoming migraine just as well as ergotamine. At the very least, marihuana reduces the duration and severity of these problems. Besides, there is often nothing else that can get my head out of the toilet when I'm vomiting uncontrollably from my always anxious stomach, migraines, or withdrawals. From repeated experience I have learned that I need both methadone and marihuana to stay off heroin. If I lack either one, I relapse.

Most antinausea drugs, muscle relaxants, antimigraine preparations, and tranquilizers hit me badly, don't work, or make the situation worse. When I was younger I used my body as a chemical waste dump. No more. Now I'm very sensitive to most drugs (except opiates, which I need in large amounts just to feel normal). In my precariously balanced, migraine-prone, opiate-addicted brain chemistry, the toxic effects of other drugs are exaggerated. Many relatively benign substances, such as the medicines mentioned above, as well as alcohol, stimulants, and sedatives, trigger withdrawal or migraine or just make me feel worse. Marihuana continues to help me as it always has, with no negative side effects. Asking me to stop taking marihuana is like telling me I can no longer stay in the program if I use Tylenol, heating pads, or ice packs.

Heroin and most other drugs clear from the urine in a couple of days, but fat-soluble marihuana can show up weeks after even secondhand exposure to the smoke. So even the most moderate, controlled medicinal use causes consistently "dirty" test results. After months of being warned to stop smoking marihuana, I was put on a thirty-day administrative detoxification. They started taking me off methadone for not being able to follow the new rules. Although no one can know how hard I tried not to, I was shooting dope [heroin] within a week.

After a couple of tearful scenes when my girlfriend caught me in the act, I made a series of desperate phone calls, following the FDA grievance procedure. I did reach one sympathetic voice, but others in the Memphis FDA office were downright hostile. The irony of this knocked me out! I knew some misinformed people felt that way about methadone, but I never expected it from the federal officials charged with overseeing the program. But then I never expected or would have believed the backward attitudes toward marihuana that have apparently taken over in our country.

Though far from sure the local courts would be any more enlightened, I even filed a lawsuit against the clinic (not feeling too good about it). Finally, at the urging of my girlfriend and a methadone advocacy group I had contacted, I arranged a transfer to the next closest methadone program, 137 miles away in Little Rock, Arkansas. Thanks to another restrictive Tennessee rule, no closer clinics are allowed.

The Little Rock program, another private clinic, accepted me, knowing the full story. Although they also (apologetically) screened for marihuana, they had regulations against forcing patients out solely on the basis of test results. But unless I gave up pot I could not have carry-out privileges. I would have to come in every day, driving halfway across the state of Arkansas. I had no choice. I would wake at 3 A.M. in the beginning of withdrawal, drive 137 miles, get dosed and counseled, turn around, and drive back. After about a month of this the Memphis clinic let me come back, but they are emphasizing that no deal is being made, and marihuana is still a problem.

I'm still hoping for the best but expecting the worst. I've put thousands of dollars, with no government help, into the only treatment that's worked, and it's hard to see how society is served by taking that from me. Maybe I am rationalizing about marihuana, but I believe common sense and science are on my side.

Most addicts have no interest in marihuana, and I wonder if some of us are long-term survivors just because we do use pot. One thing's for sure, ignoring or denying marihuana's unique medicinal effects is close-minded, blind, or worse. And sending anyone back to IV drugs for smoking pot is wrong.

MARIHUANA AND AGING

Largely by historical accident, marihuana in late twentieth-century America is regarded as exclusively a habit of the young. But it has not been so closely associated with youth at other times and places, including the United States in the nineteenth century, when cannabis was used mainly as a medicine. More than three decades have passed since marihuana first became popular in the United States, and members of the generation that learned to enjoy it then are moving toward old age. Many of them will probably discover that cannabis can ease the burdens of age as well as enhance the pleasures of youth. The people who tell their stories below may be pioneers.

James E. Dwyer, age sixty:

By comparison with some of the horrendous physical, psychological, and legal problems of other contributors to this book, my experiences with marihuana may seem mild. But I have been able to treat my health problems with it when no legal medications have been as effective. I hope an account of my experiences will prove useful to others, especially to people over fifty.

I am sixty now and discovered medical marihuana when I was forty. I had moved to Arizona, and one day, during an extremely dry period in the high desert, I overdid some physical activities and became dehydrated. This brought on a cold, and I took marihuana for the symptoms. Unlike over-the-counter cold remedies, which left me feeling mentally groggy and physically heavy, marihuana made it seem as though the cold symptoms were happening to someone else. The congestion was still there, but it was easy to ignore, and I went about my business.

In 1978 I had my first bout with influenza since leaving the Midwest. The symptoms were typical: headache, runny nose, nausea, alternating chills and fever. After several days of this I decided to light a pipeful and inhale. Within half an hour the headache disappeared, the nausea eased, and I found myself able to think about something besides the flu. Within an hour I began to feel hungry and rose from my bed to prepare a meal. I realized that the flu bug was still with me, but it didn't seem to matter. I could concentrate on work and relate to the world in my usual fashion. The flu lasted another three days, during which I inhaled whenever the symptoms became pronounced. During this illness I used no over-the-counter drugs, only fluids and marihuana.

I have also used marihuana for springtime allergies that developed after I had lived in the southwestern high desert for six years. Something about the Arizona climate—the dust, the plants, the dryness—brought on these attacks. My eyes and nose ran, and my normally high energy level was sapped to the point where all I wanted to do was lie down. I tried some prescribed allergy medications, which dried my sinuses but left me feeling drowsy. Then I switched to marihuana, and the effect was similar to my experiences with colds and flu. The symptoms abated, and I was able to stay out of bed and function normally. I kept up the marihuana treatment for a few days until all the symptoms were gone.

I have also used marihuana as a general analgesic. It dissipates most of the minor aches and pains of living past a half-century, and the ones that make it through the marihuana screen seem, once again, to be happening to someone else.

Some users say they would rather eat marihuana than smoke it because they worry about lung damage. I have known heavy marihuana smokers who suffered from dry throat, but a water pipe (hookah) usually solves that problem. I have been smoking marihuana in water pipes for twenty years without throat or lung problems.

Sometimes concern is expressed about the interactions of marihuana with other substances, such as alcohol, caffeine, nicotine, and prescribed medications. In my experience, marihuana makes an alcohol drinker lucid, a caffeine drinker calmer, a nicotine smoker less addicted, and a medication user more aware and awake. It seems to meld with whatever chemicals you ingest to make the experience friendlier. Of course, this is a matter of personal taste that should be fine-tuned over years of experience.

Another interesting combination for me has been marihuana and exercise. Especially for people over fifty, exercise is as necessary as air, food, and water to maintain a healthy, productive life. Some novice marihuana users complain that all they want to do after inhaling is lie down. But if your body feels good, marihuana will enhance that feeling, and your experiences while exercising will be rewarding. Most veteran marihuana users do not become sedentary after inhaling. They use the herb just as our ancestors did, to make physical labor bearable, even enjoyable, and to make mental labor an intriguing, even mystical adventure. I have used marihuana mostly to enjoy life more rather than to endure its pains and troubles better, but I believe that both aspects are important for senior citizens. For many older users, marihuana makes aging less of a curse and more of a blessing. By using marihuana as a general analgesic and maintaining my health through exercise and diet, I have been able to experience and understand more of life.

I have kept a careful watch for adverse effects. When I turned sixty I had a complete physical examination, including a colonoscopy, an EKG, two stress tests, and a chest X-ray. The results showed kidneys, lungs, heart, and liver working normally. Apparently twenty years of marihuana smoking has not ravaged my body, as some of our political leaders would contend.

I have learned from my experience and the experience of friends and relatives over fifty that marihuana is a highly effective, benign medication for the treatment of a variety of common ailments. It is illegal and difficult to acquire because of a political failure that needs to be addressed by our legislative bodies.

Del Brebner, age seventy-eight:

In old age it often seems that everything is depressing. "Try not to get old," I advise young checkout clerks while I'm fumbling old-lady-like for the grocery money. Sometimes I think I'm not really joking. I may make an offhand remark about the funeral of the week, but that's no joke either. At seventy-eight you attend too many funerals. The daughter of an old friend calls, and you know the instant you hear her voice that she is going to tell you that your old friend has succumbed. Of course I am reminded that I'm going to die in a minute. After all, my father died at seventy-nine.

I get an $8,000 bill from my dentist. I remember when dentist bills were around $20. My knees hurt. Why doesn't my son call? Last night I trumped my partner's ace. I've been playing pretty good bridge for sixty years, and I did that?

It is increasingly painful to observe political chicanery, corruption, and cynicism. Sophie, my best friend for seventy years, calls, and we sputter together about these things. We send newspaper editorials and columns to each other. We despair of the world.

Oh, and I forget names I have known forever. The names of friends, writers, actors, names I used this morning. I hate myself. My husband hates me too, I guess. I listen to him muttering baby talk to the cat, and I crawl into myself and feel sorry for the lost woman I was.

In short, sometimes old age seems to present a daunting parade of gloomy displeasures and discomforts. And when all these natural burdens accumulate, help is hard to get. Well, it may be easy to get Prozac or lithium. Hard to get is what may be the best medicine — marihuana. I'm trying to exercise restraint, but this is an issue on which I am tempted to moralize and preach.

An occasional hit on a simple little dried leaf in a pipe or rolled into what looks like about a third of a tobacco cigarette takes me on a small but restorative ego trip. I enjoy this three or four times a week, using about a tablespoonful of the weed altogether. The quality of the pot varies, and so do the results, but almost invariably I achieve some release from the emotional and physical burdens of a "ripe old age."

I have happy thoughts about the person whose funeral I attended recently. What fun we had together at the 1939 World's Fair! What a good life she had! All those adorable grandchildren! My father died at seventy-nine, but my mother is one hundred and two years old, and anyway, if I die I won't know it. And meanwhile I have this fabulous book to read, putting it aside now and then to prolong the pleasure. I dip up a handful of mixed nuts and munch contentedly, enjoying all those expensive bridges I paid for. My knees don't hurt. They will, but right now I don't have to go down any stairs, and anyway they're not so bad. Look at all the people who need knee surgery and hip replacement. All I have is a little discomfort. I can handle it.

I call my five-hundred-month-old baby and we share a few jokes, some news. He keeps me on the phone, and we plan a weekend. He will bring some friends I particularly enjoy. So what if I trumped my partner's ace? Don't we all do that once in a while? I'll do fine next time I play. That pension check is just dandy. It's paying for my dentist, and I don't have to put on tight shoes with heels and go to work in the morning.

Thank heaven I have Sophie to sputter with about political opportunism. We actually have a great time lashing out at our leaders. Yes, I forget names, but I almost always do well playing Famous Names, even against much younger people. And between us, my husband and I can usually come up with a name we are looking for. Hey! How can he not love me? I go over and kiss him, and together we smile down on the best cat in the world as we snuggle for a while.

I am basically an optimist, but I would have more persistent negative feelings about heading into my eighties and extinction if I did not have the pleasure of my marihuana-induced ego trips. And that's not all. I also find it helpful for insomnia, itchy skin, boredom, loss of appetite, indigestion, and—name it. Sometimes, to be sure, I recall that using the forbidden medicine is a crime, and I wonder what kind of ego trip a women's prison would provide.

Byron Stamate, age seventy-six:

I am seventy-six years old and in good health and spirits. I learned responsibility and self-reliance from my parents. I worked my way through college and served my country in World War II and for thirty years I've been an engineer and technician.

I have used and observed the use of hemp for its medicinal benefits for most of my life. My earliest recollection is from my childhood in the 1920s. Our family often visited Aunt Effie, who had severe asthma attacks. She had great difficulty breathing and became weak and distressed. When she had an attack, she would get some dried hemp leaves, crush them up, put them on a plate, ignite the hemp with a match, and place a paper cone over it. The smoke from the smoldering hemp came out of the top of the cone. I will never forget the sweet and soothing smell of the smoke as she inhaled it deeply. Her breathing was restored, and she became peaceful again. The fear and panic left all the family in the house.

In my childhood hemp was readily available in our household along with many other herbal medicines. It was used in various concoctions for the relief of numerous discomforts. My father had severe headaches from stress and overwork, and he got relief by ingesting or inhaling the smoke. Hemp is a great stress reliever. I can readily recall the smell of the hemp flowers used in cooking and baking. Hemp cookies were almost always available when necessary, and sometimes the flowers were brewed as tea. Our wise and moderate use promoted peace and tranquillity and allowed much freedom from stress and pain. As a family, we had few ills, worked hard, and were peaceful and content. All seven members of our family have been successful and in good health.

In late 1970 my wife, Frieda, was diagnosed with cancer. The cancer became painful and incapacitating and was diagnosed as terminal. The treatments were painful, ineffective, and very depressing. I recalled from my earlier years that hemp was used for relief of pain and depression and other symptoms of cancer, so we tried it. Inhaling the smoke worked well and quickly, but caused some coughing. Cooking the hemp in butter for ingesting worked well and lasted longer, but required more time to become effective and sometimes caused stomach upset. Hemp tea was not as effective but was easy and convenient to use. In spite of the difficulties, we came to the conclusion that hemp provided more comfort with less stress than any other medicine we could get. We used hemp together, and it kept both our spirits up as we were dealing with the stresses and pains of her illness. It also relieved the discomfort of my aching arthritic body. We were able to find some peace and happiness in those last few months. Frieda died in 1980.

In mid-1980 I met Shirley, and we became friends and companions. Shirley had spinal problems that caused severe back pain, leg pains, and muscle spasms. She also had periods of depression as a result of the pain. She told me she had used marihuana and it was better and more satisfactory than any other medicine that was available. Good marihuana was difficult and dangerous to get, so we grew our own. Shirley cooked it down into butter and used the green butter to make cookies. She ate one or two cookies each day to maintain a tolerable level of pain without depression. Many times, after a hard day's work constructing our country home, my stress and pain were high, and Shirley would insist that I eat a hemp cookie to get relief. Her recommendation worked, and we could share peaceful times together.

On April 5, 1990, after one year of surveillance, our privacy was violated, and we were raided by the police. I was taken to jail, and our property was seized. After one year of harassment, intimidation, and confiscation of her hemp medicine, Shirley took her own life. After forty months and over sixty court appearances, I pled guilty to cultivation charges. I was convicted of the criminal violation of supplying marihuana to my dying wife, Frieda, and to my dearest friend, the late Shirley Bell Dorsey. My acts of compassion sentenced me to be a felonious criminal, serve four months in jail, and exhaust my life savings in defense. It caused the loss of Shirley's life. I have never caused harm to anyone.

Is the present marihuana war on the good people of America proper and good for all the citizens? In review of the case against me and many other similar actions by government officials, I now ponder that question. Innocent people are being victimized, their property forfeited, lives lost, and constitutional rights denied. Costs to taxpayers have been estimated to be in the billions. Most surely there are other ways to solve the social ills that may be in America. We, the people, must demand that our sworn elected officials examine the issues and find a better way to deal with this social problem.

Few palliative medicines are available for one of the most devastating disorders of old age, Alzheimer's disease. Nineteenth-century physicians found an oral extract of cannabis to be useful. In 1890 Dr. J. Russell Reynolds wrote: "In senile insomnia, with wandering; where an elderly person, probably with brain softening . . . is fidgety at night, goes to bed, gets up again, and fusses over his clothes and his drawers; then thinks that he has some appointment to keep, and must dress himself and go out to keep it. . . . in this class of cases I have found nothing comparable in utility to a moderate dose of Indian hemp — viz., one-quarter to one-third of a grain of the extract, given at bedtime. It has been absolutely successful for months, and indeed years, without any increase of the dose." [25] Reynolds' suggestion is supported by a recent study in which Marinol was found to improve appetite and reduce disturbed behavior in patients with Alzheimer's disease. [26]

25. J. R. Reynolds, "Therapeutic Uses and Toxic Effects of Cannabis Indica," *Lancet* 1 (1890): 637–638.

26. L. Volicer, M. Stelly, J. Morris, J. McLaughland, and B. J. Volicer, "Effects of Dronabinol on Anorexia and Disturbed Behavior in Patients with Alzheimer's Disease," unpublished paper sent as personal communication.

TERMINAL ILLNESS

In the final stages of many illnesses, patients suffer increasing pain, nausea, weight loss, depression, and anxiety. Family members suffer, too, as they look on and care for the patient. Physicians try to help by prescribing a variety of medicines, but these palliatives are often ineffective, and even when they work, the side effects may be nearly as uncomfortable as the original symptoms. As the following account shows, some people are now discovering that cannabis can be extremely useful in these circumstances. Fred Hermon owns a yachting supply business in Southern California:

The effect marihuana had on my mother when she was dying of breast cancer is best described as a miracle. Mom was eighty years old at the time. We had both read extensively about the effects of cancer chemotherapy, yet we were still shocked by the savagery of the thing. She became violently ill after these treatments and would continue to vomit dozens of times daily right up to the next treatment, ten days to two weeks later. Even the smell of food cooking made her vomit. It was beginning to look as though she would die of malnutrition long before the cancer could get her. For months I listened to my mother's every breath, because I was so afraid that in her weakened condition she would choke on her own vomit and die.

Our doctor prescribed Compazine [prochlorperazine], Reglan [metoclopramide], and finally Thorazine [chlorpromazine] suppositories. Nothing worked. It reached the point where she went six full days without eating or drinking and her weight dropped to one hundred pounds. The doctor told her he'd be forced to hospitalize her and feed her through a tube in her nose. My father died in the hospital in 1974 hooked to tubes. Mom told me that if she went to that hospital and was hooked to tubes, she would never leave the hospital alive.

That's when it hit me, the memories. Back in the 1960s, I,

along with millions of other kids, smoked marihuana. I recalled how it gave me the munchies, so I asked our doctor if he had ever heard of anyone using marihuana in cases like Mom's. He said that he had and gave me his permission to try it. I got hold of some marihuana and made a little pipe out of tin foil. Mom took several puffs, and within five minutes she called out to me, "I think I can eat now." She ate for ten straight hours. Her nausea and vomiting vanished immediately.

She had her first peaceful sleep in months that night, and in the weeks after that she gained ten pounds. The staff at both clinics where she was being treated were told of the marihuana use, and they approved of it. She went completely off the standard antinausea drugs and used only marihuana from that time on. (The doctor prescribed Marinol soon after she began using marihuana, but it was ineffective, even in double dosages. It also cost more than six dollars a dose.)

Smoking turned out to be difficult for Mom, so I began adding small amounts of marihuana to her food after grinding up the leaves in a coffee bean grinder. I would add about a half teaspoonful to a special high-calorie soup, toss in a hunk or two of real butter, run it through a blender, and microwave it. A small amount of marihuana in the morning usually lasted all day. Eventually I administered even smaller amounts at intervals during the day, and this worked even better. Later I gave her the marihuana in gelatin capsules. Her only problem was getting a consistent supply of high-grade marihuana. When it ran out, her nausea and vomiting returned.

When chemotherapy ended, Mom was told she had a few weeks to several months of life left. She thought she no longer needed to use marihuana, but within twenty-four hours after stopping she began to vomit again. It was obvious that without it she would not be able to take in food and liquids. Mom lived for several months after that, and until she became comatose in the last week, she had a relatively normal life. She used those months to put her affairs in order, and I recall her telling me how happy she was to have "extra time" to be with her family. Marihuana gave her that extra time. It took away much of her pain and suffering, and, perhaps most of all, it gave her dignity. The vomiting all day and night, often vomiting all over herself, the helplessness to stop it, all that disappeared when she used marihuana. She went from dying of malnutrition and being bedridden to being able to work in her garden, visit and accept friends, eat well, and gain weight.

Near the end Mom called me into her bedroom, hugged and kissed me, and told me how thankful she was for my love and care during her illness. She said that of all the things I had done for her, providing marihuana was the best. Among her last words were, "You've got to tell people about this. You've got to let them know!" And so I have.

If there is something out there better than marihuana, medical science did not provide it, which brings up an important point. The staff at the clinics where my mother was treated approved her use of marihuana, and the clinics had bulletin boards covered with articles on cancer, but there was no mention of marihuana in these articles. My questions about this were answered with "It's a taboo subject." The horror! I knew that if it were not for my use of marihuana and my bringing up the subject, the medical establishment would never have informed our family of marihuana's life-saving effects. My beloved mother would have continued to suffer, and she would have died of malnutrition.

The scariest part of the whole story is that I had to become a criminal to obtain marihuana for medical use. It has taken me years of sacrifice and hard work to build the company I own. All that was at stake every time I got into my car and drove to a sleazy bar in a run-down section of town to buy marihuana for my mother. If I had been arrested, I would have lost my driver's license, my car, and maybe even my home. My business would have been ruined. I was Mom's sole caregiver, so she would have gone straight to a hospital. The marihuana use would have stopped, she would have been fed through a tube, and soon she would have died. Why, I ask in God's name, why? I think about this whenever I see politicians grandstanding on the marihuana issue, passing ever-tougher laws against it. God forbid they or someone they love becomes ill with cancer.

4 In Defense of Anecdotal Evidence

It is often objected, especially by federal authorities, that the medical usefulness of marihuana has not been demonstrated by controlled studies. We have already discussed the several experiments with large numbers of subjects suggesting an advantage for marihuana over oral THC and other medicines. But such studies have their limitations. They can be misleading if the wrong patients are studied or the wrong doses used. The focus of the studies is a statistically significant effect on a group, but medicine has always been concerned mainly with the needs of individual patients. Idiosyncratic therapeutic responses to a drug can be obscured in group experiments, where there is often little effort to identify the features of patients that affect responses.

Today drugs must undergo rigorous, expensive, and time-consuming tests to win approval by the Food and Drug Administration for marketing as medicines. The purpose of the testing is to protect the consumer by establishing both safety and efficacy. Because no drug is completely safe (nontoxic) or always efficacious, a drug approved by the FDA has presumably satisfied a risk-benefit analysis. When physicians prescribe for individual patients, they conduct an informal analysis of a similar kind, taking into account not just the drug's overall safety and efficacy but its risks and benefits for a given patient and a given condition. The formal drug-approval procedures help to provide physicians with the information they need to make this analysis.

First, the drug's safety (or rather, limited toxicity) is established through animal and then human experiments. Next, double-blind controlled studies are conducted to determine whether the drug has more than a placebo effect and is more useful than an available drug. As the difference between drug and placebo may be small, large numbers of patients are often needed in these studies for a statistically significant effect. Medical and governmental authorities sometimes insist that before marihuana is made legally available to patients, this kind of study should be performed for each of the indications detailed in this book.

But it is doubtful whether FDA rules should apply to marihuana. First, as we will show more fully in the next chapter, there is no question about its safety. It has been used for thousands of years by millions of people with very little evidence of significant toxicity. Similarly, no double-blind studies are needed to prove marihuana's efficacy. Any astute clinician who has experience with patients like those described in this book knows that it is efficacious to some degree for many people with various symptoms and syndromes. What we do not know is what proportion of patients with a given symptom will get relief from cannabis and how many will be better off with cannabis than with the best presently available medicine. Here large controlled studies will be helpful.

Physicians also have available evidence of a different kind, whose value is often underestimated. Anecdotal evidence commands much less attention than it once did, yet it is the source of much of our knowledge of synthetic medicines as well as plant derivatives. As Louis Lasagna, M.D., has pointed out, controlled experiments were not needed to recognize the therapeutic potential of chloral hydrate, barbiturates, aspirin, curare, insulin, or penicillin. He asks why regulators are now willing to accept the experiences of physicians and patients as evidence of adverse effects but not as evidence of therapeutic effects.[1]

1. L. Lasagna, "Clinical Trials in the Natural Environment," in *Drugs Between Research and Regulations,* ed. C. Stiechele, W. Abshagen, and J. Koch-Weser (New York: Springer-Verlag, 1985), 45–49.

There are many more recent examples of the value of anecdotal evidence. It was in this way that the use of propranolol for angina and hypertension, of diazepam for status epilepticus (a state of continuous seizure activity), and of imipramine for childhood enuresis (bedwetting) was discovered, although these drugs were originally approved by regulators for other purposes. A famous recent example is minoxidil, which was developed by the Upjohn Company to lower blood pressure. The company had no idea that topical application could restore lost scalp hair. But anecdotal evidence (later confirmed by controlled studies) was so persuasive that it is now marketed mainly as a treatment for baldness. Another drug, tretinoin (Retin-A), was originally marketed as an acne treatment. Anecdotal evidence that it had antiwrinkle properties led to formal studies proving its effectiveness for that purpose. Further studies have now been inspired by new anecdotal evidence that it can erase liver spots—brownish freckle-like blemishes on the hands and face of older people caused by exposure to sunlight.

As early as 1976 several small and methodologically imperfect studies, not widely known in the medical community, had shown that an aspirin a day could prevent a second heart attack. In 1988, a large-scale experiment demonstrated effects so dramatic that the researchers decided to stop the experiment and publish the life-saving results. On one estimate, as many as 20,000 deaths a year might have been prevented from the mid-1970s to the late 1980s if the medical establishment had been quicker to recognize the value of aspirin. The lesson is suggestive: marihuana, like aspirin, is a substance known to be unusually safe and with enormous potential medical benefits. There is one difference, however; it was impossible to be sure about the effect of aspirin on heart attacks without a long-term study involving large numbers of patients, but the reports we have presented show that cannabis often brings immediate relief of suffering, measurable in a study with only one subject. Anecdotes or case histories of the kind narrated in this book are, in a sense, the smallest research studies of all.

Anecdotes present a problem that has always haunted medicine: the anecdotal fallacy or the fallacy of enumeration of favorable circumstances (counting the hits and ignoring the misses). If many people suffering from, say, muscle spasms caused by multiple sclerosis take cannabis and only a few get much better relief than they could get from conventional drugs, those few patients would stand out and come to our attention. They and their physicians would understandably be enthusiastic about cannabis and might proselytize for it. These people are not dishonest, but they are not dispassionate observers.

Therefore, some may regard it as irresponsible to suggest on the basis of anecdotes that cannabis may help people with a variety of disorders. That might be a problem if cannabis were a dangerous drug, but, as we shall see, it is remarkably safe. Even in the unlikely event that only a few people get the kind of relief described in this book, it could be argued that cannabis should be available for them because it costs so little to produce and the risks are so small.

In addition to anecdotal evidence, there is an experimental method known as the N-of-1 clinical trial, or the single-patient randomized trial. In this type of experiment, active and placebo treatments are administered randomly in alternation or succession to a patient. The method is often useful when large-scale controlled studies are impossible or inappropriate because the disorder is rare, the patient is atypical, or the response to the treatment is idiosyncratic.[2]

Following are excerpts from an N-of-1 study published in the British medical journal the *Lancet* in 1995:

> After reading accounts in the press that smoking cannabis had improved the symptoms of other patients with multiple sclerosis, a forty-five-year-old man with multiple sclerosis persuaded his general practitioner to prescribe nabilone [the British equivalent of dronabinol]. Nabilone is a synthetic cannabinoid with powerful antiemetic effects licensed for short-term use in patients undergoing chemotherapy. He obtained immediate benefit from

2. E. B. Larson, "N-of-1 Clinical Trials: A Technique for Improving Medical Therapeutics," *Western Journal of Medicine* 152 (January 1990): 52–56; G. H. Guyatt, J. L. Keller, R. Jaeschke, et al., "The N-of-1 Randomized Controlled Trial: Clinical Usefulness," *Annals of Internal Medicine* 112 (1990): 293–299.

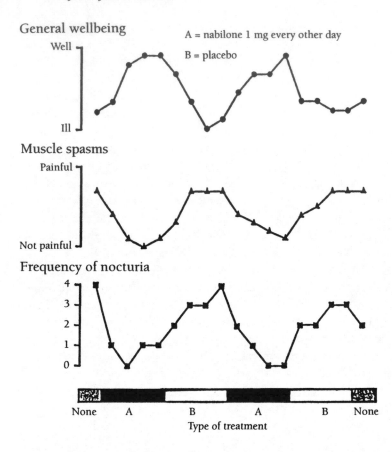

Figure 4. Symptoms of multiple sclerosis in relation to treatment with nabilone (tetrahydrocannabinol). Reproduced from C. N. Martyn, L. S. Illis, and J. Thom, "Nabilone in the Treatment of Multiple Sclerosis," Lancet 345 (March 4, 1995): 579.

a small dose of the drug, reporting decreased pain from muscle spasm, cessation of nocturia [bedwetting], and an improvement in how he felt generally. Because nabilone is only available by hospital prescription, his general practitioner was unable to continue the drug and he was referred to the Wessex Neurological Centre.

The patient had been seen . . . in 1974. At that time, symptoms and signs of right-sided sensory disturbance together with a history of uniocular central visual loss and, on fundoscopy, pallor of both optic discs suggested a diagnosis of multiple sclerosis. Over the next twenty years, his disease had pursued a relapsing and remitting course, but his disability had gradually increased. He now has a severe paraparesis [a partial paralysis of the lower limbs] and is no longer independently mobile.

We were unsure whether the improvement in symptoms that this patient reported was due to a pharmacological effect of nabilone or a placebo response and suggested to him that we evaluate the treatment in an n-of-1 trial. He readily agreed. Nabilone 1 mg every second day or placebo was given for four successive periods each lasting four weeks. The starting treatment was randomly allocated, and thereafter treatments alternated [see figure 4]. The patient knew about the design of the study, but the capsules containing nabilone were indistinguishable from those containing placebo and neither he nor his doctors were aware which treatment periods had been allocated to the active drug. He evaluated the effectiveness of treatment at the end of each week by noting frequency of nocturia on the previous night and by use of visual analogue scales to quantify pain and discomfort from muscle spasm and record how he felt generally.

The results of the trial are summarized in figure 4. The patient's reports show a striking reduction in frequency of nocturia and severity of muscle spasm and an improvement in mood and well-being that correspond to the periods of treatment with nabilone.

Transient feelings of euphoria are experienced by some patients taking nabilone. Our patient did not report such an effect, although he noticed a brief period of mild sedation after taking the active drug. This may have helped him distinguish between active drug and placebo, but it seems unlikely that the benefits he experience derived from nabilone's mood-elevating effects.[3]

3. C. N. Martyn, L. S. Illis, and J. Thom, "Nabilone in the Treatment of Multiple Sclerosis," *Lancet* 345 (March 4, 1995): 579.

Donald Spear, Greg Paufler, Robert Randall, and Harvey Ginsburg—four of the patients who tell their stories in this book—carried
out somewhat similar experiments on themselves when they alternated periods of cannabis use with periods of no use. In Paufler's case
the target symptom was muscle spasms. In Spear's case it was severe
and debilitating pruritus (itching), and in the cases of Randall and
Ginsburg, it was loss of vision. Ginsburg, as we have seen, actually
collected formal scientific data. Admittedly, in these experiments cannabis was not administered randomly in alternation with a placebo,
but the psychoactive effects of marihuana are usually unmistakable,
and few patients or observers would be deceived by a placebo. This
kind of experiment, of course, has limitations. It can be used only for
disorders that are stable and chronic, and the effect of the treatment
must be both fairly rapid and quickly reversible on discontinuation.
Nevertheless, it is certain that cannabis won its reputation as a medicine partly because many other patients around the world carried out
the same kind of experiment.

A NOTE ON THE PHYSICIAN'S ROLE

We have seen repeatedly in these case histories that people who
use cannabis as a medicine must suffer the anxiety, uncertainty, and
risks associated with obtaining and using an illegal substance. The responses of physicians, as indicated in their stories, vary a great deal. A
few are hostile or contemptuous, some are indifferent or unconvinced,
and many offer at least some encouragement or moral support. Unfortunately, most are either afraid to do more because of the law or able
to provide nothing more because they have been miseducated about
cannabis and simply know too little about its therapeutic value.

But there are also signs in these stories and elsewhere that physicians are becoming more sophisticated about this drug. As several of
the above accounts illustrate, they are learning about it in an unusual
way—not from articles in medical journals or the advertisements of
drug companies, but from their patients. In a typical case, a person
with AIDS who has been wasting away despite everything he and his

physician can do, discovers that cannabis slows down or even reverses his weight loss. On his next visit to the doctor he steps on the scale and proves it. Eventually the physician's incredulity is overcome, and he may tell other patients about it. As more and more physicians undergo this unusual form of drug education, medical societies and organizations will eventually have to change their official positions on cannabis.

That change may be on the way already. In 1995, fifty years after its editorial attacking the LaGuardia Commission, the American Medical Association invited the authors of this book to write an editorial for the *Journal of the American Medical Association*. Its title was "Marihuana as Medicine: A Plea for Reconsideration." After reviewing some medical uses of marihuana and noting its safety, we concluded: "We are not asking readers for immediate agreement with our affirmation that marihuana is medically useful, but we hope they will do more to encourage open and legal exploration of its potential. The ostensible indifference of physicians should no longer be used as a justification for keeping this medicine in the shadows."[4]

Although the journal was careful to point out that our opinion did not represent the official position of the AMA, the decision to publish it signals a change in attitude that is ultimately driven, we believe, by the experiences of patients repeatedly coming to the attention of their physicians.

---

4. L. Grinspoon and J. B. Bakalar, "Marihuana as Medicine: A Plea for Reconsideration," Commentary, *JAMA* 73:23 (June 21, 1995): 1875–1876.

5 Weighing the Risks

The benefits of any medicine must be weighed against the risks. Fortunately, there is unusually good evidence on the potential health hazards of marihuana—far better than the evidence on most prescription drugs. Not only has cannabis been used for thousands of years by many millions of people, but there is much recent research inspired by the federal government's interest in discovering toxic effects to justify its policy of prohibition. The potential dangers of marihuana when taken for pleasure and its possible usefulness as a medicine are historically and practically interrelated issues: historically, because the arguments used to justify the suppression of recreational use have had a disastrous influence on views of its medical potential; practically, because it is more likely to be safe as a medicine if it is relatively safe as an intoxicant. As the evidence makes it increasingly clear that cannabis is relatively benign, it is becoming more and more difficult to deny that a risk-benefit analysis satisfies all requirements for medical use.

The toxic effects of a drug can be classified as either acute (resulting from a single dose) or chronic (resulting from long-term use); a distinction can also be made between physical and psychological (or behavioral) effects.

ACUTE EFFECTS

The most common acute physical effects of smoking or ingesting cannabis or THC are a slight conjunctival hyperemia (reddening
of the eyes) and a slightly increased heart rate. Neither of these is uncomfortable or dangerous. Research suggests a possible explanation
for the negligible threat of cannabis to basic physiological functions:
the brain stem, which controls these functions, has few receptors for
anandamide, the natural body chemical whose effects are mimicked
by THC. After five thousand years of cannabis use by hundreds of
millions of people throughout the world, there is no credible evidence
that this drug has ever caused a single overdose death.

The lethality of drugs is ordinarily measured by a value called the
LD50, the dose that will cause death in 50 percent of the animals or
human beings taking it. The LD50 for cannabis in human beings is
not known because there are no data from which it can be derived.
The toxicity of a drug can be estimated by a number known as the
therapeutic ratio or safety factor, defined as the lethal dose divided
by the effective dose. The toxicity of THC in comparison with barbiturates and alcohol is indicated in table 2. The safety factor for secobarbital (Seconal) is 3–50 and for alcohol it is just 4–10. The safety
factor for THC, as extrapolated from data in mice, is 40,000. Many
cancer chemotherapy drugs have a safety factor of 1.5 or even less.
Marihuana in its natural form is possibly the safest therapeutically
active substance known.

Marihuana does have some acute behavioral or psychological effects
that are of concern. In some circumstances it can impair attention,
short-term memory, tracking, and coordination. There is uncertainty
about whether these effects persist for some time after the feeling of
intoxication has passed.[1] This becomes an important issue for patients

1. S. L. D. Chait, "Subjective and Behavioral Effects of Marijuana the Morning
after Smoking," Psychopharmacology 100 (1990): 328–333; J. A. Yesavage, V. O. Leirer,
M. Denari, and L. E. Hollister, "Carry-over Effects of Marijuana Intoxication on Aircraft
Pilot Performance: A Preliminary Report," American Journal of Psychiatry 142 (1985):
1325–1329. H. G. Pope, Jr., and D. Yurgelun-Todd, "The Residual Cognitive Effects of
Heavy Marijuana Use in College Students," JAMA 275:7 (Feb. 21, 1996): 521–527.

Table 2   Toxicity of THC, Barbiturates, and Alcohol

	Effective	Lethal	Safety
	Dose	Dose	Factor
Secobarbital	100–300 mg	1,000–5,000 mg	3–50
Alcohol	0.05–0.1%	0.4–0.5%	4–10
Tetrahydro-cannabinol	50 mcg/kg	2,160,000 mcg/kg[a]	40,000[a]

[a] Because no human fatalities have been documented, the figures given are for the human effective dose and the lethal dose for mice.

Source: T. H. Mikuriya, "Historical Aspects of *Cannabis sativa* in Western Medicine," *New Physician* (1969): 905.

who will be driving or otherwise operating machinery. Complex tasks requiring rapid decisions, especially in the operation of machinery, are most sensitive to the effects of psychoactive drugs. Cannabis is no exception, and people who ignore this fact may be jeopardizing themselves and others.

Opinions differ on how great the danger is. One authority states: "Clearly marihuana . . . produces serious behavioral toxicological effects. Any situation in which safety, both for self and others, depends upon alertness and capability and control of man-machine interaction precludes the use of marihuana."[2] A study of more than a thousand people treated at hospitals after accidents found that 35 percent of them had THC in their blood, 34 percent had alcohol, and 17 percent had both drugs.[3] However, THC in the blood is not a sign of cannabis intoxication, as THC (unlike alcohol, cocaine, and other drugs) may remain in the body for days or even weeks after it is ingested.

2. H. Moskowitz, "Marihuana and Driving," *Accident Analysis and Prevention* 17:4 (1985): 323–345.
3. C. A. Soderstrom, A. L. Trifillis, B. S. Shankar, et al., "Marijuana and Alcohol Use Among 1,023 Trauma Patients: A Prospective Study," *Archives of Surgery* 123 (June 1988): 733–737.

Another group of researchers has come to a different conclusion about the danger of accidents associated with cannabis:

> Several investigators have reported that marijuana reduces risk-taking propensity and driving speed. Because of these compensating tendencies, it is presently not possible to assess the net impact of marijuana as a causal agent in traffic accidents. Although some increased risk appears likely, the magnitude of the risk remains obscure. . . . Many of the laboratory studies which have shown the greatest psychomotor impairment have utilized tasks that are only abstractly related to driving. . . . It does not necessarily follow that performance on a highly novel and complex laboratory test designed to magnify performance decrements is correlated with actual "real world" performance in a vehicle. The fact that attempts to measure response to simulated accident situations have not consistently detected a marijuana-induced decrement, even at high doses, underscores the need for more research.[4]

The most careful study of this question indicated that effects of marihuana on actual driving performance were small. Compensatory concentration and effort usually overcame deficiencies caused by THC. Drivers under the influence of marihuana tended to overestimate its effects and compensated by concentrating harder and slowing down. Drivers under the influence of alcohol, on the other hand, underestimated its effects. As a result, marihuana impaired coordination less and judgment far less than alcohol did. Furthermore, the degree of driving impairment could not be predicted from the level of THC in the blood or from laboratory and roadside tests of tracking and coordination.[5] Other research shows that alcohol induces

4. R. C. Peck, A. Biasotti, P. N. Boland, C. Mallory, and V. Reeve, "The Effects of Marijuana and Alcohol on Actual Driving Performance," *Alcohol, Drugs, and Driving: Abstracts and Reviews* 2:3–4 (1986): 135–154.

5. H. W. J. Robbe, *The Influence of Marihuana on Driving* (Maastricht: Institute for Human Psychopharmacology, University of Limburg, 1994), 141, 173–176, 178.

recklessness.[6] Thus, alcohol plays a disproportionate role in accidents caused by speeding or by angry reactions to other drivers; the hazards of marihuana arise mainly from distractibility.

Doctors who prescribe anti-anxiety drugs such as diazepam (Valium) and alprazolam (Xanax) caution patients against driving, and cannabis may require similar cautions. A patient who is given 10 mg of Valium for sedation before a minor surgical procedure is forbidden to leave the hospital for some hours, and then only when accompanied. Similar precautions might be taken for people who use cannabis before cancer chemotherapy.

Two other acute "side effects" of medical cannabis must be considered. By far the most common of these is the high, or altered state of consciousness. As described by recreational users, this state lasts for two to four hours when cannabis is smoked and five to twelve hours when cannabis is taken by mouth. Its most common form is a calm, mildly euphoric state in which time slows and sensitivity to sights, sounds, and touch is enhanced. The smoker may feel exhilarated or hilarious. Thoughts flow rapidly, and short-term memory is reduced. Body image and visual perception undergo subtle changes. Often it is as though the cannabis-intoxicated adult perceives the world with some of the wonder and curiosity of a child; details ordinarily overlooked capture the attention, colors seem brighter and richer, and new values may appear in works of art that previously seemed to have little or no meaning.

As several of the people we have quoted indicate, not everyone experiences this effect, and some dislike it, but most people regard it as pleasurable and interesting. Marihuana not only relieves their symptoms but makes them feel better generally. In the words of a fifteen-year-old boy receiving chemotherapy, whose demoralizing nausea and vomiting were prevented by marihuana, "Pot turns bad things into good." We must caution the reader that this experience is exquisitely sensitive to conditions of psychological "set" (expectations and mood)

6. G. B. Chesher, "The Effects of Alcohol and Marijuana in Combination: A Review," *Alcohol, Drugs, and Driving: Abstracts and Reviews* 2:3–4 (1986): 105–120.

and social setting. In particular, descriptions of recreational use cannot necessarily be extrapolated to a medical setting.

A much less common but still significant acute psychological effect of marihuana is a state of anxiety, sometimes accompanied by paranoid thoughts and occasionally mounting to a temporarily incapacitating panic. The condition is self-limiting, and simple reassurance is the best treatment. Perhaps the main danger to the user is the possibility of being diagnosed as psychotic. There are no hallucinations, and the capacity to test the reality of thoughts and perceptions—the sine qua non of sanity—remains intact.

Anxiety and paranoid thoughts are most likely to occur in an inexperienced user taking the drug in an unpleasant or unfamiliar setting. These reactions become less common as familiarity with the drug grows. It has been noted repeatedly by government commissions studying marihuana that sophisticated users know when they have had enough and are able to titrate the dose to prevent themselves from becoming too intoxicated. In a study demonstrating this capacity, experienced marihuana smokers were given cigarettes containing no THC or 1.3 or 2.7 percent THC. When the dose was higher, they took shorter puffs and inhaled less smoke.[7]

Obviously the danger of an anxiety or paranoid reaction is magnified when the drug is illegal, its potency is unknown or uncertain, and the patient is alone and without guidance. Today even physicians who feel comfortable in recommending marihuana are sometimes ill equipped to help. The prescription of cannabis, whether through smoking or ingestion, will not be as simple as prescribing a conventional medicine. The psychoactive effects should be carefully explained so that patients will not be taken by surprise, and they may also have to learn how to recognize the effects so that they can avoid taking more than necessary. Patients who use cannabis by smoking should gain experience by taking only one puff the first time and then

7. S. J. Heishman, M. L. Stitzer, and J. E. Yingling, "Effects of Tetrahydrocannabinol Content on Marijuana Smoking Behavior, Subjective Reports, and Performance," *Pharmacology, Biochemistry and Behavior* 34 (February 1989): 173–179.

gradually increasing the number. Eventually anxiety reactions should be easy to avoid in a setting where physicians can determine the dose and prepare patients for the psychoactive effects. When cannabis is a legal medicine, patients will suffer these reactions even more rarely than they do now.

Cannabis is also sometimes said to cause an acute psychosis, described as a prolonged reaction with symptoms that include delusions, hallucinations, inappropriate emotions, and disordered thinking. The reaction is rarely reported in the United States, and given the many millions of marihuana smokers in this country, the evidence for it would be less equivocal if it occurred with any regularity. Most reports of cannabis psychosis come from India and North Africa. An authority often cited is A. Benabud of Morocco, but his description of the symptoms is far from clear; they seem to resemble other acute toxic states, including, especially in Morocco, those associated with malnutrition and endemic infections. Benabud estimates the number of kif (marihuana) smokers in Morocco suffering from psychosis as not more than five in a thousand.[8] But this is lower than the rate of all psychoses in the populations of other countries. If Benabud's estimate is correct, we would have to conclude that, if anything, marihuana protects smokers against psychosis.

A report by the American psychiatrist W. Bromberg lists thirty-one psychoses attributed to marihuana. Of these cases, however, seven involved patients already predisposed to psychoses that were only precipitated by the drug; seven others were later found to be schizophrenic, and one was later diagnosed as manic-depressive.[9] In a study examining 1,238 cannabis users in India, thirteen, or 1 percent, were found to be psychotic; this is the average rate of chronic schizophrenia in the total population of Western countries.[10] In a study conducted

8. A. Benabud, "Psychopathological Aspects of the Cannabis Situation in Morocco: Statistical Data for 1956," *Bulletin of Narcotics* 9 (1957): 2.

9. W. Bromberg, "Marihuana Intoxication: A Clinical Study of *Cannabis sativa* Intoxication," *American Journal of Psychiatry* 91 (1934): 303.

10. H. B. M. Murphy, "The Cannabis Habit: A Review of the Recent Psychiatric Literature," *Addictions* 13 (1966): 3.

by the LaGuardia Commission, nine of seventy-seven persons had a history of psychosis, but they were all patients in hospitals or other institutions. Allentuck and Bowman, the psychiatrists who examined this group, concluded that "marihuana will not produce psychosis de novo in a well-integrated, stable person."[11]

An article by V. R. Thacore and S. R. P. Shukla in 1976 revived the concept of the cannabis psychosis.[12] The authors compared twenty-five cases of what they call paranoid psychosis precipitated by cannabis to an equal number of paranoid schizophrenics. The cannabis psychotics are described as patients who developed a psychosis after prolonged abuse of cannabis. All had used cannabis heavily for at least three years, mainly in the form of bhang, the weakest of the preparations common in India. In comparison with the schizophrenic patients, the cannabis psychotics are described as more panicky, elated, boisterous, and communicative; their behavior is said to be more often violent and bizarre, and they are said to have flights of ideas without schizophrenic thought disorder. The prognosis is said to be good; the symptoms are relieved by phenothiazines, and recurrence is prevented by avoiding cannabis.

Thacore and Shukla did not provide enough information to justify the view that all these conditions were either a single clinical syndrome or related to cannabis use. They said little about the actual amount used, except that the patients' relatives regarded it as abnormally large; they did not discuss why the psychosis was associated with bhang rather than the stronger cannabis preparations. The meaning of "prolonged abuse on more than two occasions" in the case of men who were constant heavy cannabis users was not clarified, and the temporal relationship between the cannabis use and the psychosis was not specified. The cannabis-taking habits of the control group of schizophrenic patients were not discussed. It seems likely that the patients described as cannabis psychotics had a variety of syndromes,

11. S. Allentuck and K. M. Bowman, "The Psychiatric Aspects of Marihuana Intoxication," *American Journal of Psychiatry* 99 (1942): 248.
12. V. R. Thacore and S. R. P. Shukla, "Cannabis Psychosis and Paranoid Schizophrenia," *Archives of General Psychiatry* 33 (1976): 383–386.

including acute schizophrenic reactions, acute manic episodes, severe borderline conditions, and a few symptoms actually related to acute cannabis intoxication—mainly anxiety reactions and a few psychoses of the kind that may arise in unstable people under any stress or after any change in consciousness or body image.

In fact, our own clinical experience and that of others suggests that cannabis may exacerbate psychotic tendencies in some schizophrenic patients when the illness is otherwise reasonably well controlled with antipsychotic drugs.[13] Even in these patients it is often difficult to tell whether the use of cannabis is precipitating the psychosis or is merely an attempt at self-treatment for the early symptoms (needless to say, the two possibilities are not mutually exclusive). There is no reason to believe that cannabis causes or contributes to the onset of schizophrenia itself.[14]

Like many other drugs, cannabis can produce a toxic delirium when taken at very high doses, especially by mouth. The symptoms are confusion, agitation, disorientation, loss of coordination, and sometimes hallucinations. This is not a cannabis psychosis; the delirium persists only as long as large amounts of the drug are present in the brain. Unlike the delirium caused by many other drugs, it is not associated with serious physiological changes and is not physically dangerous.

One rather rare reaction to cannabis is the flashback, or spontaneous recurrence of drug symptoms while not intoxicated. Although several reports suggest that flashbacks may occur in marihuana users even without prior use of any other drug, in general they seem to occur only in those who have previously used psychedelic drugs.[15] There are also some people who have flashback experiences of psyche-

13. D. A. Treffert, "Marihuana Use in Schizophrenia: A Clear Hazard," *American Journal of Psychiatry* 135 (1978): 10.

14. G. Thornicroft, "Cannabis and Psychosis: Is There Epidemiological Evidence for an Association?" *British Journal of Psychiatry* 157 (1990): 25–33; K. T. Mueser, et al., "Prevalence of Substance Abuse in Schizophrenia: Demographic and Clinical Correlates," *Schizophrenia Bulletin* 16 (1990): 31–56.

15. V. P. Ganz and F. Volkman, "Adverse Reactions to Marijuana Use Among College Students," *Journal of the American College Health Association* 25 (1976): 93.

delic drug trips while smoking marihuana; this is sometimes regarded as an extreme version of a more general heightening of the marihuana high that occurs after the use of hallucinogens. Many people find flashbacks enjoyable, but to others they are distressing. They usually fade with the passage of time.

CHRONIC EFFECTS

In some medical uses of cannabis—for example, the relief of nausea during cancer chemotherapy—there is no need to be concerned about long-term effects. But patients who use cannabis regularly for long periods of time, as in the treatment of glaucoma, may smoke as many as ten cigarettes a day, every day. In these cases we must consider possible chronic toxic effects, both physical and psychological (or behavioral). As a result of efforts by the federal government to demonstrate the harmfulness of recreational use, there is now a vast literature on this topic. Although a study can be found to support almost any view, the findings are on the whole strikingly reassuring.

One of the first questions asked about any psychoactive drug is whether it is addictive or produces dependence. This question is hard to answer because the terms *addiction* and *dependence* have no agreed-upon definitions. Two recognized signs of addiction are tolerance and withdrawal symptoms; these are rarely serious problems for marihuana users. Beginning users actually become more sensitive to the desired effects. After continued heavy use, tolerance to both physiological and psychological effects develops, although it seems to vary considerably among individuals. Almost no one reports an urgent need to increase the dose to recapture the original sensation. What is called behavioral tolerance is probably a matter of learning to compensate for the effects of the high. It may explain why farm workers in some Third-World countries are able to do heavy physical labor while smoking a great deal of marihuana, and why glaucoma patients who smoke ten times a day can go about their lives without apparent interference from the drug. Behavioral tolerance substantially reduces the effects of intoxication on attention and motor coordination in long-term users.

A mild withdrawal reaction has been reported in experimental animals and apparently in some human beings who take high doses for a long time. The symptoms are anxiety, insomnia, tremors, and chills lasting for a day or two. It is unclear how common this reaction is; in a Jamaican study, even heavy ganja users did not report abstinence symptoms when they were deliberately withdrawn from the drug during an experiment.[16] None of the patients who tell their stories in this book suffered withdrawal symptoms when they stopped using cannabis because they feared the law or lacked the money to buy it. To the extent that a withdrawal reaction exists, it clearly does not present serious problems to marihuana users or cause them to go on taking the drug.

In a more important sense, dependence means an unhealthy and often unwanted preoccupation with a drug to the exclusion of most other things. People suffering psychological dependence on a drug find that they are constantly thinking about it, using it, or recovering from its effects. The habit impairs their mental and physical health and hurts their work, family life, and friendships. They often know that they are using too much and repeatedly make unsuccessful attempts to cut down or stop. These problems seem to afflict proportionately fewer marihuana smokers than users of alcohol, tobacco, heroin, cocaine, or even benzodiazepines, such as diazepam (Valium). Even heavy users in places like Jamaica and Costa Rica do not seem to be dependent in this damaging sense. Nerve receptors for the THC-like body substance anandamide appear to be sparse in the brain's reward center (the nucleus accumbens), where cocaine and heroin exert powerful effects. This may help to explain why cannabis is not dangerously addictive.

It is often difficult to distinguish between drug use as a cause of problems and drug use as an effect; this is especially true in the case of marihuana. Most people who develop a dependency on marihuana

16. V. Rubin and L. Comitas, *Ganja in Jamaica* (The Hague: Mouton, 1975).

would also be likely to develop other dependencies because of anxiety, depression, or feelings of inadequacy. The original condition is likely to matter more in this regard than the attempt to relieve it by means of the drug.

Much attention has also been devoted to the so-called stepping-stone hypothesis—the theory that smoking marihuana leads to the use of opiates and other dangerous drugs. In this country, almost everyone who uses any other illicit drug has smoked marihuana first, just as almost everyone who smokes marihuana has drunk alcohol first. Anyone who uses any given drug is likely to be interested in other drugs, for some of the same reasons. People who use illicit drugs, in particular, are somewhat more likely to find themselves in a company where other illicit drugs are available.

None of this proves that using one drug leads to or causes the use of another. Most marihuana smokers do not use heroin or cocaine, just as most heavy alcohol drinkers do not use marihuana. The stepping-stone metaphor suggests that if no one smoked marihuana it would be more difficult for anyone to develop an interest in opiates or cocaine. There is no convincing evidence for or against this. What is clear is that at many times and places marihuana has been used without these drugs, and vice versa.

Apart from the issues of dependence and the stepping-stone theory, the idea has persisted that in the long run smoking marihuana causes some sort of physical or mental deterioration. It would not be unreasonable to suppose that long-term use of the more potent forms of cannabis might have debilitating effects, as prolonged heavy drinking does. But the evidence is weak. One of the earliest and most extensive investigations of this question was conducted by the British government in India in the 1890s. The investigating agency, called the Indian Hemp Drugs Commission, interviewed some eight hundred persons—including cannabis users and dealers, physicians, superintendents of insane asylums, religious leaders, and a variety of other authorities—and in 1894 published a report of more than three thousand pages. The report concluded that there was no evidence that moderate use of the cannabis drugs produced any disease or mental or moral damage or that it tended to lead to excess any more than the moderate use of whiskey.[17]

In the LaGuardia study in New York City in the early 1940s, an examination of chronic users who had averaged seven marihuana cigarettes a day for eight years showed no mental or physical decline.[18] Several later controlled studies of chronic heavy use failed to establish any pharmacologically induced harm.[19] A subsequent government-sponsored review of cannabis conducted by the Institute of Medicine, a branch of the National Academy of Sciences, also found little evidence of its alleged harmfulness.[20]

These conclusions are confirmed by three major studies conducted in Jamaica, Costa Rica, and Greece. In these studies researchers compared heavy long-term cannabis users with nonusers and found no evidence of intellectual or neurological damage, no changes in personality, and no loss of the will to work or participate in society.[21] The Costa Rican study showed no difference between heavy users (seven or more marihuana cigarettes a day) and lighter users (six or fewer cigarettes a day). Studies in the United States find no effects

17. Report of the Indian Hemp Drugs Commission, 1893–1894, 7 vols. (Simla: Government Central Printing Office, 1894); D. Solomon, ed., *The Marihuana Papers* (Indianapolis: Bobbs-Merrill, 1966).

18. Mayor's Committee on Marihuana, *The Marihuana Problem in the City of New York* (Lancaster, Pa.: Jacques Cattell, 1944).

19. M. H. Beaubrun and F. Knight, "Psychiatric Assessment of Thirty Chronic Users of Cannabis and Thirty Matched Controls," *American Journal of Psychiatry* 130 (1973): 309; M. C. Braude and S. Szara, eds., *The Pharmacology of Marihuana*, 2 vols. (New York: Raven, 1976); R. L. Dornbush, A. M. Freedman, and M. Fink, eds., "Chronic Cannabis Use," *Annals of New York Academy of Sciences* 282 (1976); J. S. Hochman and N. Q. Brill, "Chronic Marijuana Use and Psychosocial Adaptation," *American Journal of Psychiatry* 130 (1973): 132; Rubin and Comitas, *Ganja in Jamaica.*

20. Institute of Medicine, *Marijuana and Health* (Washington, D.C.: National Academy of Sciences, 1982).

21. Rubin and Comitas, *Ganja in Jamaica;* W. E. Carter, ed., *Cannabis in Costa Rica: A Study of Chronic Marihuana Use* (Philadelphia: Institute for the Study of Human Issues, 1980); C. Stefanis, J. Boulougouris, and A. Liakos, "Clinical and Psychophysiological Effects of Cannabis in Long-term Users," in *Pharmacology of Marihuana,* ed. Braude and Szara, 2:659–666; P. Satz, J. M. Fletcher, and L. S. Sutker, "Neurophysiologic, Intellectual, and Personality Correlates of Chronic Marihuana Use in Native Costa Ricans," *Annals of the New York Academy of Sciences* 282 (1976): 266–306.

of fairly heavy marihuana use on learning, perception, or motivation over periods as long as a year.[22]

On the other side are clinical reports of a personality change called the amotivational syndrome. Its symptoms are said to be passivity, aimlessness, sloth, apathy, uncommunicativeness, and lack of ambition. Some proposed explanations are hormone changes, brain damage, sedation, or depression induced by marihuana. As the amotivational syndrome does not seem to occur in Greek or Caribbean farm laborers, some writers suggest that it affects only skilled and educated people who need to do more complex thinking.[23]

The problem of distinguishing causes from symptoms is particularly acute here. Some cannabis users in India and the Middle East may be hungry, sick, or hopeless and trying to soften the impact of an unbearable reality. Heavy drug users in our own society are often bored, depressed, and listless, or alienated, cynical, and rebellious. Sometimes the drug causes these states of mind, and sometimes they result from personality characteristics that lead to drug abuse. Drug abuse can be an excuse for failure or a form of self-medication. Because of these complications and the absence of confirmation from controlled studies, the existence of an amotivational syndrome caused by cannabis use has to be regarded as unproven. In fact, the only systematic examination of the relationship between marihuana use and the amotivational syndrome concluded that amotivational symptoms observed in heavy marihuana users are due to pre-existing depression.[24] This is consistent with the growing belief that some people

22. C. M. Culver and F. W. King, "Neurophysiological Assessment of Undergraduate Marihuana and LSD Users," *Archives of General Psychiatry* 31 (1974): 707–711; P. J. Lessin and S. Thomas, "Assessment of the Chronic Effects of Marihuana on Motivation and Achievement: A Preliminary Report," in *Pharmacology of Marihuana*, ed. Braude and Szara, 2:681–684.

23. W. Carter and P. Doughty, "Social and Cultural Aspects of Cannabis Use in Costa Rica," *Annals of the New York Academy of Sciences* 282 (1976): 1–16; Rubin and Comitas, *Ganja in Jamaica;* C. Stefanis, R. Dornbush, and M. Fiuk, *Hashish: Studies of Long-term Use* (New York: Raven, 1977).

24. R. E. Musty and L. Kaback, "Relationships Between Motivation and Depression in Chronic Marijuana Users," *Life Sciences* 56:23–24 (May 5, 1995): 2151–2158.

who suffer mild to moderate chronic depression find cannabis useful.

Much recent research on the health hazards of marihuana concerns its long-term effects on the body. Studies have examined the brain, the immune system, the reproductive system, and the lungs. Suggestions of long-term damage come almost exclusively from animal experiments and other laboratory work. Observations of long-term marihuana users in the Caribbean and in Greece and other studies reveal little disease or organic pathology associated with the drug.[25] For example, there are several reports of damaged brain cells and changes in brain-wave readings in monkeys after smoking marihuana, but neurological and neuropsychological tests in Greece, Jamaica, and Costa Rica found no evidence of functional brain damage. Damage to white blood cells has also been observed in the laboratory, but again, its practical importance is unclear. Whatever temporary changes marihuana may produce in the immune system, they have not been found to increase the danger of infectious disease or cancer. If there were significant damage, we might expect to find a higher rate of these diseases among young people beginning in the 1960s, when marihuana first became popular. There is no evidence of that. A large multicenter cohort study involving nearly five thousand homosexual men who were followed for eighteen months found no correlation between the use of marihuana and immune status. Furthermore, the use of cannabis had no effect on the progression of AIDS.[26]

In a 1994 study researchers found, after controlling for other factors including tobacco smoking, that HIV-positive injection drug users who also smoked illicit drugs doubled their risk of developing bacterial pneumonia (chiefly streptococcus and staphylococcus infections), from 1 percent to 2 percent per year. Nearly 90 percent of the men smoked marihuana, 26 percent snorted cocaine, and 9 percent

25. Carter and Doughty, "Social and Cultural Aspects"; Rubin and Comitas, *Ganja in Jamaica;* Stefanis, Dornbush, and Fiuk, *Hashish.*

26. R. A. Kaslow, W. C. Blackwelder, D. G. Ostrow, D. Yerg, J. Palenicek, A. H. Coulson, and R. O. Valdiserri, "No Evidence for a Role of Alcohol or Other Psychoactive Drugs in Accelerating Immunodeficiency in HIV-1-positive Individuals," *JAMA* 261 (1989): 3424–3429.

smoked crack cocaine.[27] The cause of the increased risk is unclear. Inflammatory responses might interfere with the defenses of lung tissue, or marihuana itself might become infected—a good argument for providing a regulated legal supply. Any infection is more easily transmitted when people share pipes and cigarettes—another argument for legal medical arrangements in which such sharing would be discouraged. In any case, the risk of pneumonia must be weighed against the benefits of marihuana as a treatment for the wasting syndrome. People with AIDS should be informed and allowed to choose for themselves.

Another issue is the effect of marihuana on the reproductive system. In men, a single dose of THC lowers sperm count and the level of testosterone and other hormones. Tolerance to this effect apparently develops; in the Costa Rican study, marihuana smokers and controls had the same levels of testosterone. Although the smokers in that study began using marihuana at an average age of fifteen, it had not affected their masculine development. There is no evidence that the changes in sperm count and testosterone produced by marihuana affect sexual performance or fertility.

In animal experiments THC has also been reported to lower levels of female hormones and disturb the estrus cycle. When monkeys, rats, and mice are exposed during pregnancy to amounts of THC equivalent to a human heavy smoker's dose, stillbirths and decreased birth weight are sometimes reported in their offspring. There have also been reports of low birth weight, prematurity, and even a condition resembling the fetal alcohol syndrome in some children of women who smoke marihuana very heavily during pregnancy.[28] Other studies fail

---

27. K. Waleska, D. Flahov, N. M. H. Graham, J. Astemborski, L. Solomon, K. E. Nelson, and A. Muñoz, "Drug Smoking, Pneumocystis Carinii Pneumonia, and Immunosuppression-increased Risk of Bacterial Pneumonia in Human Immunodeficiency Virus-seropositive Injection Drug Users," *American Journal of Respiratory and Critical Care Medicine* 150 (1994): 1493–1498.

28. R. Ingson, J. Alpert, N. Day, E. Dooling, H. Kayne, S. Morelock, E. Oppenheimer, and B. Zuckerman, "Effects of Maternal Drinking and Marijuana Use on Fetal Growth and Development," *Pediatrics* 70 (1982): 539–546; Q. H. Qazi, E. Mariano, E. Beller, D. Milman, W. Crumbleholme, and M. Buendia, "Abnormalities in Offspring Associated with Prenatal Marijuana Exposure," *Pediatric Research* 17 (1983): 1534.

to demonstrate any effect on the fetus or neonate.[29] The significance of these reports is unclear because controls are lacking and other circumstances make it hard to attribute causes. To be safe, pregnant and nursing women should follow the standard conservative recommendation to avoid all drugs, including cannabis, that are not absolutely necessary for their well-being.

After carefully monitoring the literature for more than two decades, we have concluded that the only well-confirmed deleterious physical effect of marihuana is harm to the pulmonary system. Smoking narrows and inflames air passages and reduces breathing capacity; some hashish smokers seem to have damaged bronchial cells. Marihuana smoke burdens the lungs with three times more tars (insoluble particulates) and five times more carbon monoxide than tobacco smoke. The respiratory system also retains more of the tars, because marihuana smoke is inhaled more deeply and held in the lungs longer.[30] On the other hand, even the heaviest marihuana smokers rarely use as much as the average tobacco smoker does. So far not a single case of lung cancer, emphysema, or other significant pulmonary pathology attributable to cannabis use has been reported in the United States.

Furthermore, the risk can be reduced. One way would be to increase the potency of the marihuana used in medicine so that less smoking would be necessary and the lungs would be less exposed to toxins. A higher potency would not necessarily heighten other dangers of marihuana because, as noted above, smokers find it easy to titrate the dose, stopping when they attain the desired effect. Another way to reduce the risk is to use various filtering and vaporizing systems, which are now foolishly discouraged by the law. If marihuana

29. P. A. Fried and C. M. O'Connell, "A Comparison of the Effects of Prenatal Exposure to Tobacco, Alcohol, Cannabis and Caffeine on Birth Size and Subsequent Growth," *Neurotoxicology and Teratology* 9 (1987): 79–85; P. A. Fried, "Postnatal Consequences of Maternal Marijuana Use in Humans," *Annals of the New York Academy of Sciences* 562 (1989): 123–132.

30. T.-C. Wu, D. P. Tashkin, B. Djahed, et al., "Pulmonary Hazards of Smoking Marihuana as Compared with Tobacco," *New England Journal of Medicine* 318 (1988): 347–351; D. P. Tashkin, B. M. Calvarese, M. S. Simmons, et al., "Respiratory Status of Seventy-four Habitual Marijuana Smokers," *Chest* 78 (1980): 699–706.

were legal, there would be strong incentives to develop further technologies for the separation of undesirable from desirable constituents
of cannabis smoke.[31]

Robert Randall, who has been smoking ten marihuana cigarettes
a day for more than nineteen years as a treatment for glaucoma, has
this to say about its medical risks and benefits:

> The power of modern propaganda is evident in the question
> seemingly intelligent people ask about my long-term use of mari-
> huana. An example: after I have spoken with a reporter for
> three hours, while cogently relating a myriad of compound facts
> in a high-density, linear, time-sensitive chronology, the reporter
> will suddenly switch subjects: "Has marihuana adversely affected
> your memory?" How can one reasonably respond to such a
> question? . . . It reminds me of the aggressive prosecutor who,
> after ranting endlessly on the hazards and horrors occasioned by
> chronic cannabis consumption, abruptly departed from his dia-
> tribe to accuse me of being a "very articulable" fellow. Articula-
> tion is, of course, the precise antithesis of scrambled synapses;
> the hallmark of a well-ordered brain at work. So one wonders
> what the prosecutor was actually asking. . . .
>
> There is a second range of questions dealing with purely
> physiologic concerns. These questions are often advanced by ado-
> lescent males who, as might be expected, favor questions relating
> to ill-disguised sexual concerns. Despite my chronic long-term
> high-dose use of marihuana, there is no gross evidence of un-
> usual breast development. I still shave at least once a day, my
> voice remains comfortably masculine, and, despite my advancing
> age, my sperm are as frisky as ever. Occasionally I even display
> profoundly territorial instincts. . . .

31. For more detailed reviews of possible deleterious effects, see L. Zimmer and J. P.
Morgan, "Exposing Marijuana Myths: A Review of the Scientific Evidence" (New York:
Lindesmith Center, 1995), a short but precise summary of the most recent literature,
and L. Grinspoon, *Marihuana Reconsidered*, 2d ed. (Cambridge: Harvard University
Press, 1978, reprinted Quick American Archives, 1994), a more leisurely examination
of the medical literature through 1977.

Of all the concerns, respiratory considerations strike me as the most obvious. We are conditioned by decades of propaganda to assume that inhaling smoke causes cancer, always. This is not, of course, the case. . . . But let us suppose this leap into the unknown is correct; that constant, long-term, high-dose marihuana use may, in some number of people, result in pulmonary or respiratory complications. What does this tell us? People with life- and sense-threatening diseases are routinely confronted by stark choices. On the one hand are the devastating consequences of a debilitating, progressive disease. On the other loom the unwanted, often highly damaging biological and mental consequences of the toxic chemicals required to check the progression of disease. This is called balancing risks and benefits. It is something all seriously ill people contend with every day of their therapy. Viewed in this medical context, marihuana is more benign and far less damaging than the synthetic toxins routinely prescribed by physicians. . . .

Marihuana has helped preserve my vision for more than fifteen years. If, with advancing age, I encounter a serious, as yet unrealized complication, such are the breaks. It is a risk I am willing to take. As W. C. Fields noted, "Life's dangerous. You are lucky to get out of it alive." In the real world, where I live, seeing is the benefit I derive from my chronic association with cannabis. On the negative side there is thankfully little to report. Nothing really. There has been no gross loss of mental capacity. There is nothing physically alarming, distressing, or even mildly annoying. . . . If confronted with a choice between vision and mental agility, agility would win. Smoking marihuana has not confronted me with such a stark choice. Instead, this humble herb has offered me many years of prolonged sight at little cost to my sanity or security.

6 The Once and Future Medicine

In September 1928 Alexander Fleming returned to his laboratory from vacation and discovered that one of the petri dishes he had inadvertently left out over the summer was overgrown with staphylococci—except for the area surrounding a mold colony. That mold contained a substance he later named penicillin. He published his finding in 1929 but the discovery was ignored by the medical establishment, and bacterial infections continued to be a leading cause of death. More than ten years later, under wartime pressure to develop antibiotic substances to supplement sulfonamide, Howard Florey and Ernst Chain initiated the first clinical trial of penicillin with six patients who suffered from a variety of infections, thus beginning the systematic investigations that could have been conducted a decade earlier.[1]

After its debut in 1941, penicillin rapidly earned a reputation as the wonder drug of the 1940s. There were three major reasons for that reputation: it was remarkably nontoxic, even at high doses; it could be produced inexpensively on a large scale; and it was extremely versatile, acting against the microorganisms that cause a great variety of diseases, from pneumonia to syphilis.

In all three respects cannabis suggests parallels:

1. G. W. Hayes et al., "The Golden Anniversary of the Silver Bullet," *JAMA* 170:13 (1993): 1610–1611.

(1) Cannabis is remarkably safe. Although not harmless, it is surely less toxic than most of the conventional medicines it could replace if it were legally available. As we have pointed out, despite its use by millions of people over thousands of years, it has never caused an overdose death. As we have also noted, the danger of lung damage can easily be addressed by increasing the potency and by developing the technology to separate particulate matter in the smoke from cannabinoids (a technology that prohibition has retarded).

(2) Medical cannabis would be extremely inexpensive. A reasonable estimate of the cost is twenty to thirty dollars an ounce, or about thirty cents per marihuana cigarette. To see what this means in practice, consider that both the marihuana cigarette and an 8 mg ondansetron pill—wholesale price, thirty to forty dollars—are effective in most cases for the nausea and vomiting most patients experience during cancer chemotherapy (although many patients find cannabis more useful). Thus cannabis would be more than one hundred times less expensive than the best legally available treatment.

(3) Cannabis is remarkably versatile. As our book has been dedicated to proving this point, we need not elaborate it here. We have reviewed the many known medical uses of marihuana, and more will undoubtedly be identified in the future.

There are also historical parallels between marihuana and penicillin. It took more than ten years to recognize the medical potential of penicillin, and its systematic exploration was long delayed by lack of interest and resources. Similarly, the urgently needed large clinical studies on cannabis have not yet begun, in this case principally because of medical indifference and government obstructionism. But just as World War II provided the impetus for research on penicillin as an antibiotic, the AIDS epidemic is now exerting pressure on researchers to explore the use of cannabis as a medicine. Initial enthusiasm for drugs is often disappointed after further investigation, but it is not as though cannabis were an entirely new agent with unknown properties. Recent research has confirmed a centuries-old promise.

As restrictions on research are relaxed and this promise is realized, cannabis may someday be recognized as the wonder drug of the new millennium.

It is distressing to consider how many lives might have been saved if penicillin had been developed as a medicine immediately after Fleming's discovery. It is equally frustrating to consider how much suffering might have been avoided if cannabis had been available as a medicine for the past two generations.

The American people are beginning to feel that frustration. There is overwhelming evidence that they think medical marihuana should be available to them. In early 1990 a scientific poll conducted by a major survey research firm for the Drug Policy Foundation, an organization working for the reform of drug laws, found that 69 percent of those polled thought doctors should be allowed to prescribe marihuana for glaucoma. A poll of one thousand representative registered voters conducted by the American Civil Liberties Union in the spring of 1995 indicates where the public stands on this issue today. Eighty-four percent of those polled thought that legalization of marihuana for medical use was a good idea, and 17 percent thought it was a very good idea. When asked the same question after being told that "conclusive tests have not been completed," 65 percent still favored legalization. Eighty-three percent thought people who found marihuana effective as a medicine should be able to use it legally. Fifty-three percent found the argument that legalizing medical marihuana would lead to more recreational use unconvincing, and 32 percent found it very unconvincing.[2]

Reformers have worked mainly within the present regulatory system to get marihuana approved as a legitimate medicine. This would be highly desirable if it could be accomplished, but it seems unlikely. The established federal system for certifying drugs is designed to regulate the commercial distribution of drug company products and protect the public against false or misleading claims about their efficacy

2. N. Belden and J. Russonello, "American Voters' Opinions on the Use and Legalization of Marijuana," survey conducted for the American Civil Liberties Union (August 1995), unpublished.

or safety. The term *drug* generally refers to a single synthetic chemical which has been developed and patented, usually by a pharmaceutical company. The sponsor submits an Investigational New Drug (IND) application to the Food and Drug Administration and begins testing, first for safety and then for clinical efficacy. When the studies are completed the company asks the FDA to approve a New Drug Application (NDA). To demonstrate effectiveness, the company is supposed to present evidence from controlled studies, not just isolated case reports, expert opinion, or clinical experience. The standards have been tightened since the present system was established in 1962. Although legal rules are technically the same, few NDAs that were approved in the early 1960s would be approved today on the basis of the same evidence. The average time for approval of an NDA is now three years.

The research is expensive, and its cost is borne by the pharmaceutical company, which may spend $200 million or more before a chemical appears on pharmacy shelves. The company will invest that large sum only if it is reasonably sure that the chemical will succeed as a medicine and the medicine will earn a profit. It has twenty years of patent protection from the date of filing to recover its investment.

Marihuana will probably never be approved by this process. One reason is that it cannot be patented. Another is that it is a plant material containing many chemicals rather than a single one (as we have noted, synthetic THC is available as a prescription drug, but most patients regard it as less effective than whole cannabis). A third reason is that marihuana is taken chiefly by smoking. No drug in the present pharmacopoeia is delivered by this route.

This is an ironical situation. More is known about the adverse effects and therapeutic uses of marihuana than about most prescription drugs. Cannabis has been tested by millions of users for thousands of years and studied in hundreds of experiments sponsored by the U.S. government over the past thirty years. It is one of humanity's oldest medicines, with a remarkable record of both safety and efficacy. Yet the FDA is legally required to classify it as a "new" drug and demand the same testing it would require for an unknown substance.

The chief justification given by the federal government for not per-

mitting medical use of marihuana is a lack of scientific studies demonstrating its efficacy. In denying the final plea for reclassification in
1992, Richard Bonner, then head of the Drug Enforcement Administration, offered the following suggestion: "Those who insist that marihuana has medical uses would serve society better by promoting or
sponsoring more legitimate scientific research, rather than throwing
their time, money, and rhetoric into lobbying, public relations cam-
paigns, and perennial litigation."[3]

Encouraged by this declaration, Donald Abrams, M.D., of the University of California at San Francisco, sought permission to conduct
a privately financed pilot study comparing high, medium, and low
doses of inhaled marihuana with dronabinol capsules in the treatment
of weight loss associated with the AIDS wasting syndrome. Abrams's
protocol was designed in consultation with the Food and Drug Administration and approved by the FDA, the University of California
at San Francisco Institutional Review Board, the California Research
Advisory Panel, and the Scientific Advisory Committee of the San
Francisco Community Consortium, which sponsored the research.

The U.S. government would not allow Abrams to obtain a legal
supply of marihuana. The Drug Enforcement Administration refused
to permit him to import it from Hortapharm, a company licensed by
the government of the Netherlands to cultivate cannabis for botanical
and pharmaceutical research. The National Institute on Drug Abuse
(NIDA), which controls the domestic supply of marihuana for clinical
research, rejected Abrams's request in April 1995. The letter of rejection was sent nine months after the request was submitted—a delay
described by Abrams and his colleagues as "unacceptably long" and
"offensive not only to the investigators but to their patients."[4] Bonner's
remark and the handling of Abrams's protocol suggest that the government has responded to the increasingly persuasive therapeutic claims

3. Marihuana Scheduling Petition, Denial of Petition: Remand, *Federal Register* 57
(1992): 10503.
4. D. I. Abrams, C. C. Child, and T. F. Mitchell, "Marijuana, the AIDS Wasting Syndrome, and the U.S. Government," Letter to the Editor, *New England Journal of Medicine*
33:10 (Sept. 7, 1995): 671.

for marihuana by urging others to investigate its medical potential and then creating obstacles that make the research impossible to pursue.

In November 1995, Representative Barney Frank of Massachusetts introduced a bill in Congress that would shift marihuana from Schedule I to Schedule II, removing one legal obstacle by declaring it to have a currently accepted medical use. FDA approval would still be required to make it a prescription drug. The prospects for early passage of the Frank bill are not bright. But even if whole cannabis somehow became available as a prescription drug, it would still be classified as having a high potential for abuse and limited medical use. Restrictions on Schedule II drugs (and all controlled substances) are becoming tighter. Nine states now require doctors to make out prescriptions for many of these substances in triplicate so that one copy can be sent to a centralized computer system that tracks every transaction involving these drugs.[5] Similar legislation is pending in other states.

In 1989 New York State added a group of Schedule IV drugs, the benzodiazepines, to the list of substances monitored in this way. The resulting surveillance of physicians has already had an effect. Research shows that many New York patients with a legitimate need for benzodiazepines are being denied them. Several reports note a rise in the prescription of substitutes that are not as safe or effective. A minimal decline in benzodiazepine overdoses has been more than balanced by an increase in meprobramate, chloral hydrate, ethclorvynol, and glutethimide overdoses. Only 6.7 percent of benzodiazepine overdoses compared to 22 percent of non-benzodiazepine overdoses were considered to be of moderate or major severity.[6]

When the DEA approved the rescheduling of dronabinol to Sched-

5. "State Multiple Prescription Programs," *State Health Legislation Report of the American Medical Association* 16 (August 1988): 35–39.

6. H. I. Schwartz, "Negative Clinical Consequences of Triplicate Prescription Regulation of Benzodiazepines," *Hospital and Community Psychiatry* 43 (April 1992): 382–385; M. Weintraub, S. Singh, L. Byrne, et al., "Consequences of the 1989 New York State Triplicate Benzodiazepine Prescription Regulations," *JAMA* 266 (1991): 2392–2397; R. S. Hoffman, M. G. Wipfler, M. A. Maddaloni, et al., "Has the New York State Triplicate Benzodiazepine Prescription Regulation Influenced Sedative-Hypnotic Overdoses?" *New York State Journal of Medicine* 91 (1991): 436–439.

ule II, it imposed some special additional restrictions that it claimed were necessary for compliance with a provision of the international Convention on Psychotropic Substances that the U.S. government has signed. This treaty mandates that parties prohibit all use of certain drugs except for scientific and "very limited" medical purposes. The DEA states its policy as follows:

> Any person registered by DEA to distribute, prescribe, administer, or dispense controlled substances in Schedule II who engages in the distribution or dispensing of dronabinol for medical indications outside the approved use . . . except within the confines of a structured and recognized research program, may subject his or her controlled substance registration to review . . . as being inconsistent with the public interest. DEA will take action to revoke that registration if it is found that such distribution or dispensing constitutes a threat to the public health and safety, and in addition will pursue any criminal sanctions which may be warranted.[7]

Ordinarily physicians are free to prescribe any drug, including those in Schedule II, for conditions and in doses other than those specifically approved by the FDA and mentioned on the product's label. Dronabinol is the only exception. It was originally approved in 1985 for the treatment of nausea and vomiting in cancer chemotherapy. More and more physicians discovered that it was useful for the AIDS weight reduction syndrome as well, and in 1992 the FDA allowed that to be added to the label. These are the only accepted uses. Thus physicians are risking their licenses to prescribe controlled substances if they provide dronabinol to a patient with any other symptoms who wishes to use a legal medicine instead of (generally more effective) whole smoked marihuana. In effect, when a patient takes dronabinol for, say, depression, instead of smoking cannabis, the legal risk is transferred from the patient to his or her physician.

When whole smoked marihuana is moved to Schedule II, the DEA will probably insist on similar restrictions. We can only specu-

7. *Federal Register* 51 (1986): 17477.

late about what might be meant by "very limited medical purposes." Would cannabis be approved for the treatment of glaucoma, epilepsy, or muscle spasms and other symptoms of multiple sclerosis? What about chronic pain and menstrual cramps? Who would decide how much depression is sufficient to justify using cannabis as an anti-depressant? And what about situations like that of Lori Horn, the patient with pseudotumor cerebri? What is she to do while waiting for systematic studies that would add her rare condition to the list of approved treatments?

In such situations physicians may be afraid to recommend what they know or suspect to be the best treatment because they might lose their reputations, licenses, and careers. Even if marihuana were available as a Schedule II drug, pharmacies would be reluctant to carry it and physicians would hesitate to prescribe it. Through computer-based monitoring, the DEA could know who was receiving prescription marihuana and how much. It could hound physicians who, by its standards, prescribed cannabis too freely or for reasons it considered unacceptable. The potential for harassment would be extremely discouraging. Unlike other Schedule II drugs, such as cocaine and morphine, cannabis has many potential medical uses rather than just a few. Many people would undoubtedly try to persuade their doctors that they had a legitimate claim to a prescription. Doctors would not want the responsibility of making such decisions if they were constantly under threat of discipline by the state. Furthermore, many doctors would not consider prescribing cannabis at all because they are victims of the government's misinformation campaign. Some still believe and promote such hoary myths as the notion that marihuana is addictive or leads to the use of more dangerous drugs.

Another problem is diversion. The cost of producing high-grade medicinal cannabis is perhaps twenty to thirty dollars an ounce, and medical distribution would add at most a few dollars more. There are about seventy marihuana cigarettes in an ounce, and the average dose is one cigarette or less. Because the government could not tax a drug used for medical purposes, medical marihuana would cost only a few cents a day. But marihuana on the street is worth its weight in gold—

$200–600 an ounce. The gap would create a powerful incentive for diversion. For all these reasons, placing marihuana in Schedule II and making it available as a prescription drug is likely to be unworkable in the long run, although important as a transitional step.

That leaves the only program now providing medical marihuana, the Compassionate IND. Since its inception, only about forty of the many thousands of patients who might benefit from medical cannabis have been approved for a Compassionate IND; as of 1996, only eight are receiving cannabis, and their supplies are often interrupted or low in quality. The government has decided not to provide cannabis to anyone else in the future. That action is cruel to the few people who might have received government cannabis, but in a broader perspective its effect is marginal and largely symbolic. The government could never have met every legitimate claim through this program without hiring a huge administrative staff, finding an army of physicians prepared to take on the heavy paperwork burden, and convincing patients that they should tolerate endless delays instead of finding marihuana on the street.

In theory, all the therapeutic properties of cannabis could be used if individual cannabinoids in addition to THC were isolated and made available separately as medicines. But this would be an enormously complicated procedure. Sponsors would have to determine the therapeutic potential and evaluate the safety of sixty or more substances, synthesize each one found to be useful, and package it as a pill or aerosol. As some of these substances probably act synergistically, it would also be necessary to look at various combinations of them. We have already explained why no drug company would provide the resources needed for such a project.[8]

8. This is not to say that individual cannabinoids might not be developed for some medical purposes. We have mentioned that cannabidiol may have some unique therapeutic properties. Resources might be found to develop it through the federal government's orphan drug program or through a use patent (one that protects a new application of a known pharmaceutical product).

Furthermore, compounds might be developed (or discovered) that act on various forms of anandamide nerve receptors, separating out the therapeutic and other effects of cannabis constituents. Already receptors for anandamide have been identified in the

Now that the anandamide receptor system has been discovered, pharmaceutical companies are searching for synthetic analogs (chemical relatives) of the cannabinoids. For example, a drug company might patent an analog that lowers intraocular pressure, can be used topically, and is free of the side effects of whole smoked marihuana. But as long as marihuana itself is available, the company might have difficulty earning a profit on that drug. They might have to price it so high that many would prefer to buy or grow marihuana instead. This has already proved to be true of Marinol in many cases.

In 1992 the Maine legislature passed a bill that would have become law but for the governor's veto. Under this bill marihuana would have been distributed to pharmacies, and physicians approved by a special review board would have had the right to prescribe it to patients who were (1) being treated for glaucoma or undergoing chemotherapy for cancer, (2) in danger of going blind or dying, and (3) not responding to conventional treatment or suffering severe side effects from conventional treatment.

Although modeled in part on the state programs of the 1970s and 1980s, the Maine proposal went further. First, it would have allowed citizens to defend themselves under state law against criminal charges of marihuana cultivation or possession by showing that they had a diagnosis of glaucoma or were suffering from serious nausea or vomiting from cancer treatment. Second, the "therapeutic research program" established by the law would have been allowed to use marihuana confiscated by local police if NIDA refused to supply it.

In November 1996, the voters of California approved an initiative that allows patients and their caregivers to possess and cultivate marihuana if they are using it on the recommendation of a physician for the treatment of "cancer, anorexia, AIDS, chronic pain, spastic disorders, glaucoma, arthritis, migraine, or any other illness for which mari-

---

spleen, a major organ of the immune system, and have proved to be of a different type from those found in the brain. See S. Munro, K. L. Thomas, and M. Abu-shaar, "Molecular Characterization of a Peripheral Receptor for Cannabinoids," *Nature* 365 (Sept. 2, 1993): 61–65.

huana provides relief." The initiative also provides that no physician will be punished or sanctioned for recommending marihuana. The passage of this legislation may be a milestone in the history of marihuana as a medicine, if only for what it reveals about public opinion.

It is a disadvantage as well as an advantage that the referendum refers to many rather than just a few narrowly defined medical uses. The breadth of the language could create problems that lead to the intervention of the federal government. In the same month the voters of Arizona, by a two-thirds majority, approved a more restrictive initiative that would allow doctors to prescribe Schedule I drugs, including marihuana, to seriously or terminally ill patients. Physicians would be required to get a second written medical opinion approving the prescription, and they would have to document scientific research supporting their use of the drug. In general, such legislation is difficult to implement because it threatens to bypass the federal regulatory system, and the federal government is unlikely to allow its authority over drugs to revert to the states. The legislation may, however, provide a defense for medical marihuana users who are arrested.

Although laws like the the vetoed Maine bill and the California and Arizona initiatives may not offer a long-term solution to the problem of medical marihuana, they are signs of a growing public restiveness about the present laws. If similar proposals are adopted in several other states, the federal government will face a political challenge, a needed debate will ensue, and the public will be made aware of the importance of the issue.

Shortly before the federal government closed down the last legal avenue of access, people in need of medical marihuana began to organize and supply it to one another in open defiance of the law by establishing cannabis buyers' clubs, beginning in San Francisco in 1991. There are now several of these clubs in cities around the country. The clubs buy cannabis wholesale and supply it at or near cost to patients who have a written note from a doctor. A typical club is the Green Cross Patient Co-op, located in the Seattle area. The operators describe it as "open to all that present a bona fide need for medicinal cannabis on the advice of their physician or other health care professionals."

CANNABIS
BUYERS'   CLUB
CINCINNATI OHIO

PHYSICIAN STATEMENT

My patient _____

is suffering from _____.

We have discussed the medicinal benefits of cannabis usage as a therapy for this condition. We have discussed the risks associated with his/her decision to use cannabis as a treatment for this condition. I would consider prescribing cannabis for my patients condition if I were legally able to do so. If my patient chooses to use cannabis therapeutically, I will monitor his/her condition and provide advice on his/her progress.

_____

Signed

_____

Dated

_____

Physician's Name

_____

Address

_____

City, State, Zip

Figure 5. Physician statement form, Cannabis Buyers' Club, Cincinnati, Ohio.

Patients fill out and sign a membership application on which they are asked to state their symptoms, the medications they are now taking, and the uses and side effects of marihuana. The patient's doctor signs a Physician Statement (figure 5). Patients are asked to make a donation to cover the price of the marihuana they buy and the operating costs of the co-op. Those who cannot pay may receive the marihuana free.

Until early 1995, state and federal governments were reluctant to close down buyers' clubs for fear of hostile public reactions. The first serious action against open suppliers of medical marihuana was taken in the spring of 1995, when police raided the Green Cross Patient Co-op. One of the co-op's directors, Joanna McKee, is confined to a wheelchair and has severe muscle spasms that she treats with marihuana. She served a two-day jail sentence in August 1995, after leaving the state against the orders of a judge to attend a NIDA conference on marihuana in Washington. The charges against Green Cross were dropped after a judge disallowed the search warrant used for the raid. Johann Moore, the head of the Underground Cannabis Buyers' Club in New York City, and Richard Evans, of the Greater Cincinnati Cannabis Buyers' Club, were arrested in 1996. The charges against Moore were dropped; Evans served a month in prison for "trafficking" marihuana within 1,000 yards of a school, although of course he was not supplying it to children. In August 1996, the San Francisco Buyers' Club, the nation's oldest and largest, with nearly 10,000 members, was closed down by state narcotics agents under the direction of the state Attorney General, despite the vigorous objections of the San Francisco city government. Buyers' clubs have also been raided in Key West, Florida, and in Los Angeles, but many others, including the Green Cross Patient Co-op, continue to function.

The persistence and growth of these clubs are a sure sign that medical marihuana has the approval of increasing numbers of Americans. More and more patients will undoubtedly join buyers' clubs as they learn from word of mouth and experience that marihuana may relieve their symptoms. It appears that, in effect, in addition to prescription and over-the-counter pharmacy sales, a third, illegal set of institutions is being formed for the distribution of this medicine. But because buyers' clubs are and will almost certainly remain illicit, they are vulnerable to corruption, diversion of marihuana, and attacks by the authorities. They may play an important transitional role in bringing the benefits of medical cannabis to the attention of the public, but they can never serve more than a fraction of those who might find cannabis useful. They are not a permanent solution to the problem of medical accessibility.

Given that cannabis is such a remarkably safe, versatile, and effective medicine and could be a remarkably inexpensive one if the prohibition tariff were eliminated, why is the U.S. government so adamantly opposed to any arrangement that would legalize it? At least three reasons come to mind:

(1) The government has been exaggerating the dangers of recreational marihuana for almost seventy years. It has spent many millions of dollars in efforts to demonstrate some harm that would justify prohibition. Since 1967 more than ten million Americans have been arrested on marihuana charges, and many of them have had to serve long prison sentences. Careers have been ruined and families bankrupted or destroyed. The damage is beyond estimation. It is difficult for the government to turn around now and say, "Sorry, we made a mistake." Governments don't readily acknowledge mistakes.

(2) There are now considerable vested interests in maintaining prohibition. The drug war has created a vast enforcement and "educational" bureaucracy, a drug-abuse industrial complex that parallels the military-industrial complex produced by the Cold War and is just as difficult to unseat. Forfeitures of drug dealers' property fill the coffers of the drug-control system, supplemented by the illegal seizures of corrupt drug agents. The drug war juggernaut also sustains a growing industry devoted to examining the hair and urine of citizens for traces of marihuana and other drugs. The pharmaceutical companies and drug-testing laboratories that profit from this practice do not want to see it end. Meanwhile, a mirror-image industry on a smaller scale develops techniques for defeating the drug tests and markets them through such magazines as *High Times*. Illicit marihuana dealers of course also profit from the present system, and so do the people

who provide hydroponic lighting and control equipment to growers who seek safety from the law by moving indoors. All in all, a large and growing investment of capital and human resources is involved.

(3) Finally, marihuana has become a symbol charged with cultural tensions. Along with psychedelic drugs, it was seen as a catalyst of the antiestablishment movement of the 1960s and 1970s. Many regarded the free speech, civil rights, and anti–Vietnam War movements as socially healthy and exciting expressions of a vibrant democracy. But others saw these movements as symptoms of a society out of control —just look at how those marihuana-smoking young people dressed and wore their hair! Even today, culturally conservative people are fearful of marihuana, and the media play to their fear by presenting marihuana users as deviant. Successful middle-class users passively cooperate with this campaign when they keep their use secret and allow the media to focus on latter-day hippies.

There is a century of history behind the legal and institutional obstacles erected against medical marihuana. Like cannabis, most psychoactive drugs that are now severely restricted by law have had significant medical uses at some places and times. These drugs have tended to fall into disuse as their dangers are more strongly emphasized, other treatments become available, and governments place more controls on the practice of medicine. The history of social and legal responses to the use of these drugs provides many examples of hypocrisy, corruption, inadequate pharmacology, inconsistent responses based on inadequate information, indulgence of various social prejudices in response to drug scares, and institutional self-aggrandizement by drug enforcement agencies. But there is a worldwide trend more significant than any of these details.

All nations have similar drug laws, which are supplemented by international treaties and drug control agencies. In the nineteenth century in the United States and Europe there were almost no government controls on drug use. The growth of manufacturing, capitalist entrepreneurship, and the spirit of liberal individualism made that period an age of self-medication and competing medical authorities. Almost anyone was free to sell almost anything as a medicine. The patent medicine industry flowered, and many of its products contained psychoactive drugs, including alcohol, opium, and cocaine. Orthodox physicians used these drugs, too, and hospital pharmacies stocked large amounts of wine. As late as 1910 morphine was estimated to be the fourth most commonly used medicine, and alcohol was fifth.[9] Distinctions among categories of use were not clear. Often there was little practical difference between a person drinking in a nineteenth-century saloon and someone taking a "tonic" that contained alcohol as its main active ingredient.

Some of the psychoactive drugs, like much strong medicine, could also be powerfully poisonous. Their dangers (as well as their effectiveness) were magnified by isolation of the active chemicals in pure form and the development of such technologies as the hypodermic syringe, which permitted intravenous and intramuscular injection. Mistrust of these drugs had begun to grow by the beginning of the twentieth century. They had been used freely without a careful distinction between medical and other purposes—an ambiguity that now began to seem dangerous.

Advances in the art and science of medicine paralleled these developments. The rise of synthetic chemistry, experimental physiology, and bacteriology created hope for a scientific medicine based on the recognition of specific disease agents for specific diseases. But the psychoactive drugs were not specific cures; they relieved suffering in many situations, but a pharmacologically inactive nostrum occasionally did the same. The powers of the drugs began to seem indeterminate and uncontrollable—more reliable than quack medicines, but no less dangerous and mysterious. By the early twentieth century the idea was becoming common that these were subtle poisons with intrinsic powers of deception. Even the best-informed person could be possessed by them, becoming dependent or addicted. Taking cocaine to feel alert or opiates to relax could no longer be legitimated as a medical treatment. These drugs were subjected to strict worldwide

9. M. C. Smith and D. A. Knapp, *Pharmacy, Drugs, and Medical Care* (Baltimore: Williams and Wilkins, 1972), 61.

criminal controls, and nonmedical cannabis use was banned in many American states. Even alcohol was criminalized for more than a decade, and its status as a medicine was permanently lost.

The new restraints imposed beginning at the turn of the century resulted from an impulse to clean up society, impose classifications, and reduce disorder. Just as physical hygiene required government measures to prevent infectious disease, and professional hygiene required higher standards for medical and pharmaceutical practice, it seemed that intellectual hygiene required clear and enforceable categories for the use of psychoactive drugs. The process that began with restrictions on patent medicines eventually affected even the power of individual physicians to prescribe psychoactive drugs. Controls were placed on the manufacture and distribution of these substances; certain medical uses were carefully defined, and almost all other uses were outlawed.

In the United States the federal government assumed the control of psychoactive drugs through the Pure Food and Drug Act (1906), the Harrison Narcotics Act (1914), and the Volstead Act (1919). Although the ban on alcohol was repealed in 1933 under intense public pressure, the system has otherwise persisted, and it has been further elaborated in a series of laws leading up to the Comprehensive Drug Abuse Prevention and Control Act of 1970 and its successors.

All this was part of the process by which nineteenth-century liberal capitalism transformed itself into a state corporate system. At the same time the organized medical and pharmaceutical professions, sometimes in collaboration with drug·companies, consolidated their power, incorporating more and more social functions in a process that has been labeled by hostile critics "medical imperialism." In what is now known as the Progressive Era, the Pure Food and Drug Act, the Harrison Narcotics Act, and the Volstead Act were characteristic legislation as much as the Federal Reserve Act, which reformed the banking system.

Government control over nonpsychoactive therapeutic drugs grew at a slower pace and in a different way, but the trend toward centralization and restriction is similar, and the assumption too is similar: that free individual choice in this field is becoming largely pointless because it is illusory. Of all federal laws, only the Pure Food and Drug Act of 1906 was designed to encourage free choice because it was aimed at simple fraud—mislabeling. Federal restrictions on non-psychoactive drugs began with the Food, Drug, and Cosmetics Act of 1938. That law was amended in 1962 to establish the New Drug Application (NDA) system, under which the federal government has the power to decide which drugs will be legally available to physicians. The decision had been made that even doctors need protection from misinformed or inappropriate uses of drugs. It was entirely consistent with this view for the DEA to argue in the marihuana rescheduling case that even widespread approval by physicians was not enough to justify making marihuana legally available as a medicine.

The greatly increased complexity of the pharmacopoeia explains some of the changes that have occurred since the end of the nineteenth century. Free individual choice seemed more justifiable at a time when the average consumer might be thought to have almost as good a claim as anyone to evaluate the safety and usefulness of the few available medicines. It is more plausible to say in the present situation that consumers and even physicians can no longer know enough to make that judgment for themselves, and only authoritative scientific knowledge can supply the basis for decisions.

The system of control over nonpsychoactive drugs is based on this consumer protection model. It is a powerful justification for government control because it usually applies to areas of social life in which individual autonomy seems least valuable. The principle is that in a complex society far more needs to be known than any single person can learn, and that there are some things about which the average person cannot make an informed and rational choice without prior safeguards. Under this system, drugs without accepted medical uses can be seen as resembling defective and therefore dangerous machines or toys. Drugs with medical uses are useful as instruments for certain purposes, but only with safeguards to be supplied by manufacturers and distributors under government direction.

Medical regulations are quite properly the strictest of the consumer protection laws because the dangers involved can be so great, and the seemingly reliable intellectual authority of science supports any regulatory system. A medical definition of drug control provides a stay against confusion and has therefore become important in public thinking. In a poll conducted in the early 1970s, 30 percent of those who were asked to choose the best of several definitions of drug abuse chose "use for nonintended purpose, nonmedical use" (27 percent chose "excessive use").[10] We expect the rules against taking risks in medicine to be stricter than the rules against taking risks in the pursuit of pleasure, wealth, or ambition. If an activity as dangerous as professional boxing came under medical control, it would certainly be banned, as the American Medical Association wishes.

But even this control system has been considered inadequate for psychoactive drugs. Prohibition of so-called narcotics began long before prescriptions were legally required for ordinary drugs. The government was telling doctors that using opiates to maintain addicts was not a legitimate medical practice for many years before it started to substitute its judgment for that of physicians about the availability of nonpsychoactive drugs. This regime of highly restrictive controls continues. Something more than consumer protection is involved when the laws criminalize even the consumer and require a vast police bureaucracy for their enforcement. We do not fine or jail the patients of someone who practices medicine without a license or the customers of a manufacturer who disobeys consumer protection laws, yet the mere possession of cannabis and other illicit psychoactive drugs is a federal crime. The metaphor of war is rarely invoked in the name of consumer protection but constantly used in the assault on psychoactive drugs. The reason is that laws controlling these drugs are ultimately aimed not at consumer protection but at containing what is believed to be a threat to the social fabric and moral order. If the social fabric and moral order are at stake every time someone casually uses a drug, we need no subtle arguments about whether people need to be protected from themselves.

10. National Commission on Marihuana and Drug Abuse, *Drug Use in America: Problem in Perspective* (Washington, D.C.: U.S. Government Printing Office, 1973), 12.

Yet this distinction is never clearly made because a certain conception of public health seems to include both purposes. Psychoactive drug use evokes the image of a plague or epidemic possibly more often and more powerfully than any other social problem. That image suggests a moral crusade that is also a public health campaign. The imagery of disease has tremendous social potency; it eliminates most moral and political doubts. Stopping an epidemic of typhoid presents no moral problems, so why should stopping an epidemic of drug abuse? Concerns about individual freedom become irrelevant. Preventing disease has been regarded as a government responsibility for more than a century. National and international systems for the control of psychoactive drugs developed along with international institutions devoted to preventing the spread of infectious disease. Here the government acts even on remote and indirect possibilities of harm, as when it requires vaccinations. The vocabulary in which we talk about psychoactive drug use permits a smooth transition from physical and psychological to moral and finally to social health. Consumer safety and morality, amalgamated through references to health and disease, reinforce one another as justifications for control.

When talking about the dangers of nonmedical drug use, we tend to use the broadest possible definition of health in order to justify the strongest restrictions; for example, we prefer to put more weight on the indeterminate notion of social well-being than on concrete and specific physical health problems. In establishing legitimate purposes for using drugs, of which health is obviously one, we define health narrowly, so that again severe restrictions can be justified. Protecting, preserving, or enhancing well-being in a broad sense is regarded as a legitimate reason for banning drugs, but not as a legitimate reason for using them.

But we are much more likely to disagree about threats to the health of a moral or social order than about threats to individual physical (or even psychological) health. Individual values differ, and causes are difficult to distinguish from symptoms in such issues as public tranquillity or productivity. As a result, public consensus is weak, and the laws may seem arbitrary. Common sense on this issue may be nothing more than shared prejudice. Attitudes toward minorities, work, worldly success and failure, sex, and family life may be the real issues in a controversy about drugs. The government insists on viewing marihuana as a threat to society, but the very need to use the rhetoric of war may be a sign that the issue is not settled; obviously, many people doubt whether this war is worth fighting.

Moral consensus about the evil of cannabis is uncertain and shallow. We pretend that eliminating drug traffic is like eliminating slavery or piracy or eradicating smallpox or malaria. No one would suggest that we legalize piracy or give up the effort to eradicate infectious diseases. Yet the economist Milton Friedman and the editors of the *National Review* and the *Economist* of London, among many others, have come to believe that we should legalize marihuana and other drugs. The official view is that everything possible has to be done to prevent anyone from ever using any controlled substances. But there is also an informal lore of drug use—marihuana use above all—that is far more tolerant. Many of the millions of cannabis users in this country not only disobey the drug laws but do not acknowledge the laws' moral authority. Some users are ambivalent, some are hypocritical, and some are in open or secret resistance. The people who tell their stories in this book do not conceal their bitter resentment of laws that make them criminals. They believe that they have been deceived, and they have come to doubt that the "authorities" understand much about either the deleterious or the useful properties of marihuana.

Furthermore, the costs of prohibition are high and rising. In 1995 nearly 600,000 people were arrested on marihuana charges alone— the highest number in American history.[11] Governments at all levels now spend many billions of dollars a year on drug enforcement and on the housing and feeding of drug dealers and users in local jails and state and federal prisons. One-third of federal prisoners are now confined on drug charges, many of them on marihuana charges. Drugs enter the United States at a growing rate despite the war effort, which

11. "Crime in the United States: 1995," *FBI Uniform Crime Reports* (Washington, D.C.: U.S. Government Printing Office, 1996), 207–208.

only inflates prices and keeps the franchises of dealers lucrative. Crime and violence are now produced by the black market in drugs, as they were produced by the black market in alcohol in the 1920s. Civil liberties are eroded by the use of informers and entrapment, mandatory urine testing, and unwarranted searches and seizures. Young people who discover that the authorities have been misleading them about cannabis become cynical about their pronouncements on other drugs and disdainful of their commitment to justice. The resulting undercurrent of ambivalence and resistance in public attitudes creates room for the possibility of change.

Meanwhile, the confinement of psychoactive drugs (except alcohol) to medical contexts is being increasingly questioned. The doctrine of specific etiology, based on infectious and dietary deficiency diseases, is the source of modern medicine's great triumphs, and yet it remains inadequate. For the vaguely defined functional problems that still account for many visits to doctors, we often still have no clear explanations and no better remedies than drugs that affect the mind and senses.

This situation naturally causes much unease. Doctors are accused by laypeople and accuse one another of using pills to resolve problems of living that demand more complex and difficult adjustments. On the other hand, there remains a large area in which diseases and problems of living overlap. Often a doctor's prescription of a tranquilizer is not very different from a layperson's self-prescription of a beer or a marihuana cigarette—just as an alcohol-laced tonic often fulfilled the same function as whiskey in the nineteenth century.

In any discussion of drugs it can be difficult to draw a line between therapeutic and recreational uses or between normalizing and enhancing uses. The controversy about the significance of the popular antidepressant fluoxetine (Prozac) illustrates this problem. Drug use has been assigned to various social categories, including magic and religion as well as medicine and, recently, self-enhancement. In preindustrial societies distinctions among these categories are not always clear. In these societies medical diagnosis and prognosis have an aura of the occult, and disease is often considered an instrument of gods or evil spirits. The words *health* and *holiness* have a common root, meaning "whole." Because modern industrial societies consider it important to keep these categories separate, they have difficulty in regulating and controlling the use of psychoactive drugs.

It has become so important for modern societies to limit the purposes for which drugs are used that they have a tendency to be suspicious of any proposal that leaves those purposes ambiguous or vague. Modern restrictions on what qualifies as religion make it difficult, for example, to allow drug use for religious purposes. But we must learn to live with that ambiguity if we are to use drugs in ways that best promote the development of human powers. In some contexts that may mean rejecting the sharp distinction between medical and other uses.

In the case of cannabis, it is becoming increasingly clear that the demand for legal enforcement of that distinction is incompatible with the realities of human need. Marihuana use simply does not conform to the conceptual boundaries established by twentieth-century institutions. It enhances many pleasures and has many potential medical uses, but even these two categories are not the only relevant ones. The kind of therapy often used to ease everyday discomforts does not fit any such scheme. In many cases what laypeople do in prescribing marihuana for themselves is not very different from what physicians do when they supply prescriptions for psychoactive or other drugs.

Consider the following case: a ninety-two-year-old woman with severe congestive heart failure, hypothyroidism, cerebral artery insufficiency, and glaucoma (among other maladies) complained of insomnia. Her doctor was reluctant to add one more potent medicine to the eight she was already receiving (in the form of twenty-five pills a day), so he suggested that she have a glass of wine at bedtime—not a conventional solution, but one that was fairly safe and in this case proved to be effective. Here the doctor was acting like a nineteenth-century physician in treating alcohol as a therapeutic substance. In the nineteenth century he could have recommended one or two minims of a tincture of cannabis for the same purpose. Today, alas, that is impossible, although marihuana might be safer and more effective.

Marihuana is also used in a quasi-medicinal way to enhance creativity and productivity. A common problem in the treatment of manic-depressive disorder with lithium carbonate is the complaint of patients that the medication robs them of some of their creativity, vitality, and enjoyment of life—one reason so many of them stop taking it even though they know the potentially disastrous consequences. Mild mood elevation (hypomania) often enhances creative thinking, and experiments show that a better mood often produces more original associations and creative problem-solving. Speed of thought and an easy flow of ideas are associated with elevated mood in bipolar patients.[12] Curiously, these are also common features of cannabis intoxication. In the following account a forty-two-year-old health professional explains how she uses marihuana both to enhance creativity and to make continued use of lithium possible—another situation in which medical and nonmedical uses are impossible to separate.

In my late twenties, while pursuing an undergraduate degree in the medical sciences, I began to experience the debilitating effects of bipolar affective disorder, commonly known as manic depression. For almost ten years I denied the problem and avoided seeking treatment because of a deep-seated irrational fear: I was unwilling to acknowledge mental illness in myself because my father had been hospitalized for schizophrenia most of his adult life. But eventually my physical and mental health began to deteriorate. I had longer depressions and more severe manic episodes; my social and professional life suffered seriously. At the age of thirty-four I realized that I had to face up to my problem, sought treatment, and recovered with the help of lithium carbonate and psychotherapy. Since then I have faithfully taken lithium and have stayed in remission while continuing to grow personally and professionally.

Marihuana has also played an important part in my recovery and continued remission. I started using it regularly in my middle twenties, at about the time I entered college. In my late twenties I moved away from the college community and no longer had

12. K. R. Jamison, "Mood Disorders and Patterns of Creativity in British Writers and Artists," *Psychiatry* 52 (May 1989): 125–134.

access to marihuana. Within a few weeks I realized how helpful it had been in relieving some symptoms of my (still unacknowledged) mood disorder. During episodes of hypomania I feel unpleasant tension in all my skeletal muscles; marihuana relaxed those muscles more effectively and with fewer side effects than alcohol. Luckily, I was able to gain access to marihuana again and resumed using it, taking two or three puffs two or three times a day.

My psychiatrist asked me to stop using marihuana and gave me a prescription for Xanax (alprazolam) instead. To maintain control, I took as little as I could, just as I had done with marihuana. Xanax worked, but it had undesirable side effects such as dry mouth and sedation. I continued to use marihuana as well, although I now smoked it only once or twice a week. I stopped using Xanax as soon as the lithium took effect.

After my recovery I returned to school and earned an advanced degree in my medical profession. By now, like many people with bipolar disorder, I was noticing that lithium prevented not only hypomanic mood swings but also the state of consciousness associated with creativity. I feared losing my creativity for both personal and professional reasons. I pursue artistic hobbies for relaxation, and my work also benefits greatly from creative insights—for example, recognition of meaningful patterns in diverse data or new perspectives on obstinate problems. For that reason I continue to use marihuana moderately. I smoke it from a small pipe; usually two or three puffs last me three to four hours. Marihuana allows me to attain the creative state of mind that is so precious to me without having to stop taking lithium and risk a relapse. I also continue to find it useful as a muscle relaxant, especially in treating menstrual cramps.

The following story illustrates in still another context the relationship between medical and nonmedical uses:

How do I, a seventy-three-year-old retired-to-the-country woman, happen to be a casual marihuana smoker? Simple. What I read and heard in the sixties (when I was in my forties) per-

suaded me to try it. I simply could not believe that all those in-
telligent young people (including my son) were doing something
stupid and destructive. Of course many were, but not, I think, in
smoking marihuana. When a friend and contemporary, a musician, offered to introduce me to reefer madness I accepted. That
was—imagine!—a quarter of a century ago.

I have been smoking marihuana in all those twenty-five years,
sometimes daily, sometimes occasionally. I smoke it because I
enjoy the incredible comprehension of music, the heightened
perception of color and form, the diminishment of current problems and pressures, the extension of time. If having an hour and
Twinkies with funny friends feels like four hours and gourmet
food, do I have to go to jail?

As important as the pleasure, though, is what seems to me
to be a palliative quality to marihuana. In an accident twenty
years ago I suffered two or three broken ribs. Medical advice was
to leave 'em alone, they'll come home. At the time I was employed as editor and operations coordinator of a federally funded,
university-based education project. All day long I worked hard,
lugging books and printouts and instructional materials up and
down, and all day long I suffered excruciating pain from the broken ribs. I would go home at night, have a couple of tokes on
a joint, and, pain-free or at least pain-unaware, I would enjoy a
few hours with people, go to bed, and sleep. Yes, for me, if I want
it to be, marihuana is Halcion. Funny?

Currently I am troubled by itchy eyes and face. I have seen
three doctors and two dermatologists, the second of whom is
certain that I suffer from a contact dermatitis. He has embarked
on a search for the allergen. So far I have had cortisone cream
(in varying strengths) prescribed three times. This may well be
a degenerative condition. Whatever it is, when I am seriously
uncomfortable and the cortisone seems to be insufficient, a few
tokes of the smoke of a mild green plant and the itch is not gone
but of no concern to me. For this do I pay a ten-thousand-dollar
fine, lose my home, and go to jail?

One more thought on this medicinal application of marihuana: My father, deceased, and my mother, ninety-eight, both had glaucoma. Considering my gene pool, might I be a likely candidate for the disease? I know nothing about the dosage or source of marihuana used in glaucoma therapy, but it occasionally crosses my mind that my longtime recreational use of marihuana may have been helpful in protecting me from developing glaucoma.

Through all the years that I have engaged in criminal behavior, including growing a few evil plants, I have maintained a successful career in writing and teaching writing. My own published work, in addition to uncountable reports, news releases, proposals, etc., includes a respectably published, enthusiastically reviewed novel and several stories and articles in such publications as *Woman's Day* and *McCall's*. Over these same years I have continued my own writing and taught writing and advertising in a junior college and a major university. I have maintained a home, entertained guests, taken full care of my mother for several years, taken care of children from time to time, and gained a reputation as a gourmet cook. (I'm not; I simply follow good recipes precisely.) What I am trying to indicate is that my use of marihuana has never been a drain on my productivity or effectiveness. It has only enhanced my enjoyment of life and, as indicated above, helped me through some medical difficulties.

A musician describes his use of marihuana for creative purposes:

Over the years marihuana has served as a creative stimulant to my work as a performer and my more occasional inspirations as a composer. Almost all my choral pieces and songs have been composed partly or wholly under the influence: melodic and rhythmic ideas just pop into my head during relaxed and happy moments—"points of creative release"—and these seminal ideas are formed into a whole composition over a period of days to years.

Marihuana has also helped me as a performer to gain insights into the meaning of musical masterpieces. Practicing new repertoire while using marihuana is not a good idea, since the keen mental concentration needed to learn notes is somewhat impaired. But once I have learned a piece fluently, marihuana enhances my understanding of what it means as an entirety.

On an average practice day, I work in the morning after drinking a few cups of coffee. In the late afternoon I often have a little workout in the gym, then come back to the piano, smoke some marihuana, and practice enjoyably and productively for one or two hours. I never try to perform in public while stoned, but I often listen to music after smoking marihuana, as do many other musicians I know.

I recently saw a television special on the life of Louis Armstrong in which his lifelong affection for marihuana was pointed out. He found it both an inspiration for his music and a balm against life's trials. It works the same way for me; it's one of my best friends (although I prefer to take it in another form than smoking).

A scientist reports on the contribution of cannabis to his work:

As a scientist I have spent years training the analytical side of my mind. I have learned to be suspicious of my data, to look for ways to test the reasonableness of my results and arrive at the same conclusions by alternative means. It is an active process of mental discipline: idealizing physical situations, making assumptions to formulate a soluble problem, and applying logic to determine the outcome.

What I have sometimes neglected is an awareness of the wider significance of my work and the sense of wonder that led me into the field to begin with. Often I have been unable to see an answer that lies before me. Part of the blame lies in the very training that enables me to do complicated analytical work. To concentrate on the aspects of a problem that I have included in my model, I ignore apparent distractions that sometimes hold the key to a solution. This happens especially when I work with computers, which can do nothing with the mere suggestion or hint that something important has been left out. It is a human habit to go over old ground repeatedly, seeing what you believe to be there rather than what is actually there (the reason people cannot proofread their own writing). I get high for short periods to remedy this problem. It allows me to turn off the rational side of my mind and think creatively (and randomly). It temporarily cancels the limiting effects of my training and allows me to see my work in a different light.

It would be inefficient to follow up these new ideas while high because I am too easily distracted and my analytical capacity is impaired. Instead I enjoy the relaxation and keep notebooks recording my thoughts in lists and outlines. Both the relaxation and the observation of otherwise overlooked details have been valuable contributions to my work.

Another scientist who has found cannabis useful tells his story:

I am a forty-year-old geologist who studies the surfaces of planets and moons at a National Aeronautics and Space Administration research center. I began smoking marihuana in high school, partly out of curiosity and partly in response to peer pressure, after observing no ill effects on my friends who used it regularly. Since then I have used it for self-exploration, for religious experiences, and, of course, for pleasure, including enhanced appreciation of sex, music, art, and conversation. But cannabis has done more than that for me; it has actually helped me to acquire a professionally useful skill.

To analyze the underlying structures and history of geological change on a planet or moon, planetary geologists rely on images of landforms and surface markings radioed back from spacecraft. Landforms cannot be understood unless they are perceived in three dimensions by means of stereo images — paired photographs taken from slightly different angles to mimic depth perception.

Most people use mechanical devices — stereo-opticons of one sort or another — to judge depth from stereo photos. The machinery needed to view stereo images of planetary surfaces is particularly awkward and time-consuming to use. A few fortunate people can see three dimensions in stereo photographs without mechanical aids—a skill every planetary geologist would like to have.

When I was an undergraduate, a friend tried for months without success to teach me this skill, and I became convinced that people who said they possessed it were deluding themselves. But one evening we smoked some especially potent marihuana, purely for pleasure. I amused myself by looking at a pair of stereo photographs that had been left in the room. Suddenly the two pictures merged into a single three-dimensional view. It was like a gift from God. Overjoyed, I looked at other stereo pairs and discovered that I could perceive depth in them as well. I spent the rest of the evening gazing at stereo pairs. The next day, when the immediate marihuana effects had passed, I found that I retained the ability. The skill has saved me a great deal of time in consulting and analyzing stereo photos of geological field sites.

I believe my experience illustrates how marihuana can overcome deep conditioning, initiated immediately after birth, that locks us into perceiving reality in very narrow and formulaistically defined ways. Marihuana shares with its stronger psychedelic brethren the power to cleanse the doors of perception and make the world seem as new. Its help in catalyzing the acquisition of a skill useful in my work is only one of the many blessings and insights it has provided.

There is no longer any doubt that cannabis has useful properties that cannot be described as medical. It can be an intellectual stimulant, helping users to penetrate conceptual boundaries, achieve fluidity of associations, and enhance insight and creativity. Some find it so useful in gaining new perspectives or seeing problems from a different vantage point that they smoke it in preparation for intellectual or creative work. Other nonmedical uses of cannabis have less to do with learning. It can enhance appreciation of food, sexual activity, natural beauty, and other sensual experiences, and it can bring a new dimension to the understanding of music and visual arts. Under the right conditions and in the right settings, it can promote emotional intimacy. For almost everyone it has the capacity to highlight the comical in life and catalyze a deep and salutary laughter.

The criminalization of marihuana use in general and the policies that make marihuana legally unavailable as a medicine are two problems with the same cause and the same solution. Marihuana is caught in a dual web of regulations—those that control prescription drugs in general, and the special criminal laws controlling psychoactive substances. These mutually reinforcing laws establish a set of social categories that strangle its medical potential. Whatever interim measures we may decide to take, ultimately we will have to cut the knot by giving cannabis the same status as alcohol—legalizing it for all uses and largely removing it from the medical and criminal control systems.

Opponents of medical marihuana sometimes say that its advocates are insincere and are only using medicine as a wedge to open the way for recreational use. Anyone who has studied the history of desperate efforts to obtain legal marihuana for suffering people knows that this is untrue. The attitude falsely ascribed to medical marihuana advocates is actually a mirror image of the government's own attitude. The government is unwilling to admit that marihuana can be a safe and effective medicine largely because of a stubborn commitment to wild exaggeration of its dangers when used for other purposes. Far from believing that medical availability of marihuana would open the way to other uses, we take the view that the regulated availability of cannabis under the same rules applied to alcohol may be the only way to make its judicious medical use possible. As we noted earlier, cannabis conclusively lost its medical status as an almost incidental effect of the Marihuana Tax Act of 1937, which was designed to prevent "recreational" use. The full potential of this remarkable substance, including its full medical potential, will be realized only when we end that regime of prohibition established two generations ago.

Index

Abdominal mesothelioma, 39
Abrams, Donald, 257
Acetaldehyde, 202
Acetaminophen (Tylenol), 109, 110, 120,
    121, 122–123, 126, 130–131, 135,
    171, 175
Acetazolamide (Diamox), 51, 60, 192
ACLU. See American Civil Liberties
    Union
ACTH (adrenocorticotropic hormone),
    80, 82–83, 87, 90
Adapin (doxepin), 147
Addiction (drug), 243–245, 268; heroin,
    210–212; marihuana as treatment for,
    6, 11, 206–210; opiates, 210–212;
    opioids, 109, 210; tobacco, 11, 209,
    216. See also Alcoholism
Addiction (marihuana), 7, 8–9, 11, 48,
    58–59, 243–245
Adrenocorticotropic hormone. See ACTH
Adriamycin (doxorubicin), 23, 24, 40,
    41
Advil, 171
Africa, 3, 240
Aggression, 11. See also Violence
Aging, 214–221
AIDS, 22, 100–109, 248, 254, 262; AIDS
    wasting syndrome, 21, 102, 232–233,
    249, 257, 259; and IND applications,
    21, 22

Alcohol, 59, 269; and depression, 207–
    208; interactions with, 109, 216; as
    medicine, 87, 268, 275; research on,
    101, 235–236, 237–238
Alcoholism, 11, 202–210, 244
Alkeran (melphalan), 23
Allentuck, Samuel, 11, 210, 241
Allergies, 215
Alliance for Cannabis Therapeutics, 15,
    21
Alprazolam. See Xanax
Alzheimer's disease, 221
American Civil Liberties Union (ACLU),
    255
American Medical Association, 8, 9, 12,
    233, 271
American Society of Clinical Oncology,
    45
Amitriptyline (Elavil), 119, 139, 143,
    148, 184
Amphetamine, 143
Amsterdam, 107
Analgesic properties, 3, 4, 6, 7, 97, 111,
    215
Analgesics, 14, 109, 110, 127, 200
Anandamide, 3, 235, 244, 261–262n,
    262
Anecdotal evidence, 13, 163, 226–233
Anesthetic effects, 5, 173
Angina, 228

Ankylosing spondylitis, 129–131
Anorexia, 262
Anslinger, Harry, 7–8, 11, 195
Antabuse (disulfiram), 202
Antacids, 184
Antibiotics, 172
Anticonvulsant properties, 67
Anticonvulsants, 141, 201
Antidepressant properties, 97. *See also*
    Depression
Antidepressants, 139–140, 149–150,
    201, 202, 205
Antiemetics, 24–25, 28, 33, 40, 229
Antihistamines, 127
Antimicrobial effects, 172
Antipsychotic drugs, 178, 181, 242
Antisocial behavior, 11
Antitumoral effects, 173
Anxiety, 5, 178, 245; side effect, 19, 44,
    55, 239–240
Appetite: loss, 21, 139, 175, 189, 218;
    stimulation, 3, 5, 11, 98, 101–102,
    103, 168. *See also* AIDS; Cancer
    chemotherapy
Arizona, 263
Armstrong, Louis, 280
Arrests: and buyers' clubs, 265; for cul-
    tivation, 21–22, 54, 62, 63, 65–66,
    74, 75, 78–79, 99, 134, 195, 207,
    220–221; for possession, 104, 117–
    118, 136–137, 185, 193. *See also*
    Criminalization; DARE
Artane (trihexyphenidyl), 175
Arthritis, 127–129, 262
Arthur D. Little Company, 13
Asia, 3
Aspirin, 7, 76, 109, 125, 127, 131, 171,
    175, 184, 227, 228
Asthma, 5, 6, 164–167, 219
Ataxia, 88–89, 91, 94
Ativan (lorazepam), 175
Atopic dermatitis, 131–135, 146. *See also*
    Skin disorders
Atropine, 105
Attention deficit disorder (ADD), 176–
    178

Azathioprine (Imuran), 87, 170
AZT (Zidovudine), 21, 101, 104, 105,
    106

Baclofen (Lioresal), 80–81, 90, 94,
    95–96, 100
Barbiturates, 7, 106, 107, 143, 210, 227,
    235–236
Benabud, A., 240
Benzodiazepines, 81, 201, 244, 258
Beta-agonists, 164, 165
Beta-blockers, 46, 63, 66, 124
Betaxolol, 63
Betoptic, 63
Bhang variety, 2, 241
Bipolar disorder. *See* Manic-depressive
    disorder
Birch, E. A., 210
Birth weight, 249. *See also* Childbirth
Bladder control, 4, 90–91, 97, 98, 100
Bone cancer, 27, 43
Bonner, Richard, 257
Bosiger, Collin, 196–198
Botulinum toxin, 174, 175
Bouquet, R. J., 11
Bowel control, 91
Bowman, Karl M., 11, 210, 241
Brain, 2–3, 118, 248, 262n
Breast cancer, 41, 222
Brebner, Del, 217–219
Bromberg, W., 240
Bronchitis, 5
Bronchodilators, 164
Brookhiser, Richard, 36–39
Bupropion (Wellbutrin), 148, 159
Bureau of Narcotics and Dangerous
    Drugs (BNDD), 13–14
Burke, James, 42
Burns, 172
Burton, Richard, 3
Bush administration, 22, 186
Buspar (buspirone), 147
Buyers' clubs. *See* Cannabis buyers' clubs

Calcium, 111
Calcium channel blockers, 124

California, 262, 263, 265
California Research Advisory Panel, 257
Campaign Against Marihuana Production (CAMP), 78, 79
Cancer, 27, 110, 173, 219–220, 248, 252, 262. *See also specific forms of cancer*
Cancer chemotherapy, 18, 23–45, 78, 118, 229, 259, 262; side effects of drugs used in, 23–24, 30, 40, 222, 235
Cannabidiol, 2, 44, 68, 167–168, 176, 178, 179–181, 261n
Cannabidiolic acid, 172
Cannabinoids, 2, 164, 165, 173, 178, 229, 254, 261, 261n. *See also* Congeners: cannabinoid; THC
Cannabinol, 2, 173
Cannabis, 1. *See also* Marihuana
Cannabis Action Network, 200
Cannabis buyers' clubs, 263–266
Cannabis Corporation of America, 15
Canter, Murphy, 170–171
Carbamazepine (Tegretol), 67, 141, 153
Carbonic anhydrase inhibitor, 46, 51
Caribbean research, 247
Carisoprodol (Soma), 175
Carteolol (Ocupress), 66
Cass, Chuck, 208–209
Centennial Exposition (1876), 4
Cerebral artery insufficiency, 275
Cervical dystonia. *See* Dystonias
Chang, Alfred, 43
Charas variety, 2
Chemotherapy. *See* Cancer chemotherapy
Childbirth, 3, 5, 249. *See also* Birth weight; Labor pains
Children's Hospital (Boston), 111
China, 3
Chloral hydrate, 7, 210, 227, 258
Chlorambucil (Leukeran), 23
Chlordiazepoxide, 184
Chlorpromazine, 124. *See also* Thorazine
Cimetidine (Tagamet), 184
Cisapride (Propulsid), 189, 190

Cisplatin (Platinol), 23, 28, 36, 37, 38
Clinical trial methods, 229–232
Clonazepam (Klonopin), 67, 100
Clorazepate (Tranxene), 74
Cocaine, 10, 236, 244, 245, 248–249, 260, 268
Codeine, 100, 110, 120, 122, 124, 125
Cognitive effects, 3, 7, 41
Colds, 127, 214
Cold sores, 172
Committee on Cannabis Indica, 4
Compassionate Use IND. *See* Investigational New Drug: Compassionate Use
Compazine. *See* Prochlorperazine
Compound Q, 104
Comprehensive Drug Abuse Prevention and Control Act (1970), 13, 15, 16, 269; Schedule I drugs, 13, 16, 263; Schedule II drugs, 13, 106, 107, 258–261; Schedule III drugs, 16, Schedule IV drugs, 14, 258
Congeners: of THC, 7, 67; cannabinoid, 13, 27, 262. *See also* Dronabinol; Levonatradol; Nabilone; Synhexyl
Congestive heart failure, 275
Constipation, 3
Controlled Substances Act. *See* Comprehensive Drug Abuse Prevention and Control Act
Convention on Psychotropic Substances, 259
Convulsions, 5
Corral, Valerie, 76–80
Corticosteroids, 80, 87, 131, 186, 191
Cortisone, 132, 188
Costa Rica, 244, 246, 248, 249
Coughs, 4
Council on Mental Health, 13
Cramps, 127, 135–137, 260, 277
Creativity, 275–276, 277, 279–281, 282
Crime, 11, 274
Criminalization, 8, 283; and cost of marihuana, 21–22, 61, 144, 194–195, 260, 271; and difficulty of obtaining marihuana, 23, 59, 150, 171, 223,

Criminalization (continued)
232; dilemma of, 30–31, 35, 52–
54, 71–72, 96, 105, 106–107, 135,
152–153, 155, 156–157, 185–186,
190–191; and drug testing, 199; and
fear of arrest, 30–31, 35, 71, 78, 147,
157, 166, 175, 224–225, 232; pro-
hibition tariff, 41, 43, 266; results
of, 221, 266–267, 273–274. See also
Arrests; DARE
Crohn's disease, 186–188
Culpeper, Nicholas, 4
Curare, 227
Cyclophosphamide (Cytoxan), 23–24
Cyclosporine, 170
Cylert (pemoline), 177
Cytomegalovirus retinitis, 108
Cytoxan (cyclophosphamide), 23–24

Dantrolene (Dantrium), 81
DARE (Drug Abuse Resistance Educa-
tion), 158, 159
Darvocet, 122–123
Darvon (propoxyphene), 98, 122, 125,
184
Davis, J. P., 67
Decongestants, 127
Demerol (meperidine), 59, 98, 124, 125,
127, 211
Depakote (valporic acid), 67, 141, 153
Dependence. See Addiction (drug);
Addiction (marihuana)
Depression, 3, 6, 11, 127, 138–150, 168,
178, 245, 247
Dermatitis, 131–135, 146, 278. See also
Skin disorders
DeRopp, R. S., 12
Desert Storm syndrome, 198, 199
Desipramine (Norpramin), 139, 147,
149–150
Desyrel (trazodone), 92, 148, 175
Dexamethasone, 119–120, 121
Dexedrine (dextroamphetamine), 101,
143
Diabetic gastroparesis, 189–191

Diamox (acetazolamide), 51, 60, 192
Diana, Sam, 85–86
Diazepam. See Valium
Digestion, 3, 5
Dilantin. See Phenytoin
Dilaudid. See Hydromorphone
Dingell, John, 9–10
Diphenoxylate, 105
Diphenylhydantoin sodium. See Phe-
nytoin
Dipivefrine (Propine), 63
District of Columbia Court of Appeals,
17
District of Columbia Superior Court, 57
Disulfiram (Antabuse), 202
Diuretics, 191
Dosage: potency of, 192; titration of, 39,
43, 44–45, 108, 152, 154, 239, 250
Doxepin (adapin), 147
Doxorubicin (Adriamycin), 23, 24, 40,
41
Dronabinol, 14, 43–44, 178, 257, 258–
259. See also Congeners; Marinol
Drug abuse, 271
Drug Abuse Resistance Education. See
DARE
Drug companies, 255–256, 262, 269
Drug Enforcement Agency (DEA), 14–
17, 20, 21, 62, 257, 258–260, 270.
See also Bureau of Narcotics and
Dangerous Drugs; Federal Bureau of
Narcotics
Drug Policy Foundation, 13, 255
Drug testing, 199, 266, 274
Drug war, 266–267
Duborg, George, 168–170
Dwyer, James E., 214–216
Dysentery, 3
Dysmenorrhea, 5, 6
Dystonias, 174–176

EAE. See Experimental autoimmune
encephalitis
Ear infections, 172
Economist (London), 273

Ecotrin (aspirin), 125
ECT. See Electroconvulsive treatment
Edinburgh New Dispensary (1794), 3
Elavil. See Amitriptyline
Electroconvulsive treatment (ECT), 150
Emphysema, 250
Endometriosis, 102, 137
England, 4
Ephedrine, 125, 165–166
Epilepsy, 4, 6, 66–80, 260
Epinephrine (adrenaline), 46, 51
Ergotamines, 124, 212
Erythromycin, 170
Estrus cycle, 249
Ethclorvynol, 258
Ethiopian Zion Coptic Church, 15
Ethosuximide (Zarontin), 67
Europe, 3, 4
Evans, Richard, 265
Expectorants, 127
Experimental autoimmune encephalitis (EAE), 94
Experiments, 27, 229–232, 248

Fasulo, Teresa, 187–188
FDA. See Food and Drug Administration
Federal Bureau of Narcotics, 7, 8, 12
Fentanyl, 175
Fetal alcohol syndrome, 249
Fetus, 249–250
Fevers, 3
Fine, Benjamin, 50, 53, 56, 57
Finnegan-Ling, Deborah, 200–202
Fix, Judy, 135–137
Florida, 22, 62, 117, 118, 265
Fluorouracil, 41
Fluoxetine. See Prozac
Food and Drug Administration (FDA), 16, 17, 18–19, 27, 77, 102, 213, 258, 259; and drug-approval proce-dures, 226–227, 256, 257; and IND program, 20–21, 22, 62, 116–117, 118
Food, Drug, and Cosmetics Act (1938), 270

Foscarnet (Foscavir), 108
Frank, Barney, 258
Frei, Emil, 25, 27
Friedman, Milton, 273

Galen, 3
Ganja variety, 2, 244
Gindlesperger, Greg, 193–195
Ginsburg, Harvey J., 63–66, 232
Glaucoma, 18, 45–66, 232, 243, 251, 255, 260, 262, 275, 279
Glutethimide, 258
Gonorrhea, 5. See also Venereal diseases
Gould, Stephen Jay, 39
Granisetron (Kytril), 24
Greater Cincinnati Cannabis Buyers' Club, 265
Greece, 246, 247, 248
Green Cross Patient Co-op, 263, 265
Grinspoon, Danny, 25–27
Grinspoon, Lester, 13, 25, 119–150, 190
Gulf War syndrome, 198. See also Desert Storm syndrome

Haldol (haloperidol), 179–181, 198
Hanson, Gordon, 72–76
Hare, H. A., 5
Harrison Narcotics Act (1914), 10, 269
Hashish, 2, 4
Headaches, 3, 219. See also Migraine
Hemp, 1, 3, 4, 5. See also Marihuana
Hepatitis B, 103
Herbal healing and medicines, 125, 175
Hermon, Fred, 222–225
Heroin, 210–212, 244
Herpes, 172
HIV (human immunodeficiency virus), 101, 104, 248
Hodgkin's disease, 32
Hokanson, Russ, 97–99
Horn, Lori, 191–193, 260
Hortapharm, 257
Human immunodeficiency virus. See HIV
Hutchins, Joe, 182–186

Hydrocodone, 175
Hydromorphone (Dilaudid), 112, 113, 118, 175, 211
Hyperemesis gravidarum, 168
Hypertension, 171, 228
Hypnotic properties, 3, 5, 6, 7, 98, 167–168
Hypomania, 276, 277
Hypothyroidism, 111, 275

Ibuprofen, 109, 131, 135, 192
Ifosfamide (Ifex), 23
Imipramine (Tofranil), 139, 145, 149, 184, 228
Imitrex (sumatriptan), 124
Immune system, 94, 248, 262n
Imuran (azathioprine), 87, 170
Incontinence, 4. See also Bladder control; Bowel control
IND. See Investigational New Drug
India, 2, 3, 4, 195, 240, 241, 245, 247
Indian Hemp Drugs Commission, 245
Influenza, 215
Insomnia, 6, 61, 97, 139, 167–168, 175, 178, 218, 275
Institute of Medicine, National Academy of Sciences, 246
Insulin, 227
Intermittent Aggressive Disorder, 196
International Cannabis Research Society, 201
International Chiefs of Police, 15
Investigational New Drug (IND), 17, 18–19, 20, 21; application process, 20–21, 62, 86, 116, 256; Compassionate Use, 20, 22, 58, 63, 86, 186, 261; Individual Treatment, 20
Isocarboxazid (Marplan), 139
Isoproterenol, 164–165, 167
Isoxsuprine (Vasodilan), 184

Jaffe, Norman, 27
Jamaica, 244, 246, 248
Jenks, Kenneth, and Barbra Jenks, 21

Johns Hopkins University: Wilmer Eye Institute, 56
Johnson & Johnson, 42
Jules Stein Eye Institute (UCLA), 55

Kane, H. H., 202–203
Kaolin, 105
Kidney failure, 168–170
Kleber, Herbert D., 22
Klonopin (clonazepam), 67, 100
Kuala Lumpur (Malaysia), 196
Kuhn, Paul, 41
Kytril (granisetron), 24

Labor pains, 137–138
LaGuardia, Fiorello, 11
LaGuardia Commission, 11–12, 210, 233, 241, 246
Lamivudine (3TC), 108
Lasagna, Louis, 227
Latanoprost (Xalatan), 46, 66
Law(s), 93, 204, 216, 250–251, 255, 267, 273; Arizona, 263; California, 262, 263; federal, 269–270; Maine, 262, 253; Michigan, 32
Lawn, John, 17
Lee, Kay, 127–129
Legalization, 254, 258–261, 262
Leifer, Ron, 148–150
Leukemia, 25, 78; acute lymphatic, 26
Leukeran (chlorambucil), 23
Levonatradol, 2
Librium, 132, 145, 184
Lioresal. See Baclofen
Lithium carbonate, 127, 140, 143, 146, 148, 150, 152–156, 158, 159, 161, 162, 217, 276–277
Longcope, James C., 168
Loperamide, 105
Lorazepam (Ativan), 175
Louisiana, 18
Lung cancer, 250
Lungs, 248. See also Pulmonary system

Maine, 262, 263
Malaria, 3
Malaysia, 196
Manic-depressive disorder, 139, 140,
150–162, 240, 276–277
Marihuana: botanical classification, 1;
chemical compounds, 2; compared
to tobacco, 250; geographic distribution, 1, 2, 3; government supply
of, 19; industrial uses, 1, 8; potency,
2, 19, 21, 102, 117, 118, 241, 250,
254; smoked vs. oral THC, 20, 43–45,
47, 226; and tolerance, 11, 47, 202,
243–244, 249. *See also* Side effects
Marihuana Tax Act (1937), 7, 8, 11, 283
Marinol, 262; and AIDS, 102–103, 105,
107–108; and alcoholism, 206, 207;
and Alzheimer's, 221; and cancer,
36, 45, 223; and depression, 149,
150; and glaucoma, 55; and nausea,
169–170; and pain, 201, 202. *See also*
Congeners; Dronabinol
Marplan (isocarboxazid), 139
Mason, James, O., 22
Mason, Ron, 103–105
Massachusetts, 17, 185
Mattison, J. B., 6–7, 209
Mayo Clinic, 113
McKee, Joanna, 265
McLemore, Alan, 203–207
MDMA. *See* 3,4-methylenedioxy-
methamphetamine
Medical necessity defense, 22, 57, 65,
185, 263
Medical use: criteria for, 15–16; decline
in, 7–8. *See also specific diseases and
conditions*
Megace (megestrol acetate), 102
Melancholia, 141
Melorheostosis, 122
Melphalan (Alkeran), 23
Memphis, 211
Menstruation, 5. *See also* Cramps; Dys-
menorrhea; Premenstrual syndrome

Meperidine. *See* Demerol
Meprobamate (Miltown), 145, 258
Merritt, John, 57
Mesalamine, 186, 188
Methadone, 175, 211–213
Methaqualone (Sopor), 112, 113, 118
Methocarbamol (Robaxin), 175
Methotrexate, 41
Methylphenidate. *See* Ritalin
Methysergide, 124
Metoclopramide (Reglan), 189, 190, 222
Mexico, 2
Michigan, 29, 31–32; Marihuana as
Medicine Bill, 32
Middle East, 2, 3, 247
Midol, 127
Migraine, 6, 123–126, 169, 212, 262.
See also Headaches
Miller, Carol, 124–126
Miltown (meprobamate), 145, 258
Minoxidil, 228
Miotics, 46
Missouri, 17
M'Meens, R. R., 5
Monoamine oxidase (MAO) inhibi-
tors, 139–140. *See also* Isocarboxazid
(Marplan); Phenelzine (Nardil);
Tranylcypromine (Parnate)
Moore, Johann, 265
Moreau de tours, Jacques-Joseph, 141
Morocco, 240
Morphine, 6, 116, 175, 209–210, 260
Motrin (ibuprofen), 192
MS. *See* Multiple sclerosis
MS Contin (morphine), 175
Mudrane, 125
Multiple congenital cartilaginous exosto-
sis, 111–118
Multiple sclerosis (MS), 80–94, 229,
231, 260
Muscle relaxant(s), 113, 212; marihuana
as, 4, 212, 277
Muscle spasms, 3, 88, 93, 94, 100, 232,
260, 265

Music appreciation, 278, 281, 282
Musikka, Elvy, 58–63
Musty, Richard E., 200
Mysoline (primidone), 67, 72, 73, 74, 76

Nabilone, 2, 229–231
Naproxen, 131
NAPT pills (nerve gas antidote), 199
Narcotics, 106, 107, 109, 210
Narcotics Commission of the League of Nations, 11–12
Nardil (phenelzine), 140
National Academy of Sciences, 246
National Cancer Institute, 18, 43, 113
National Eye Institute, 55
National Federation of Parents for Drug-Free Youth, 15
National Institute of Drug Abuse (NIDA), 19, 21, 62, 118, 257, 262
National Institutes of Health (NIH), 113
National Organization for the Reform of Marijuana Laws (NORML), 13–15, 54, 167, 185
National Review, 273
Nausea: and AIDS, 21, 102–103, 105, 106; and cancer chemotherapy, 18, 19, 24–30, 33–35, 36–39, 40, 41–42, 43–44, 78, 222–224, 259; and other causes, 168–171, 189
Negen, Deborah, 32
Neonates, 249–250
Neoplasms, 101
Nerve gas antidote (NAPT pills), 199
Nervous system, 189
Netherlands, 257
Neuralgia, 5, 6
Neuroleptic drugs, 176
New Drug Application (NDA), 256, 270
New English Dispensatory (1764), 3
New Mexico, 17, 18–19
New York City, 11, 265
New York state, 258; Department of Health, 20
Nitrogen mustard derivatives, 23, 24

Nonsteroidal anti-inflammatory drugs. See NSAIDs
NORML. See National Organization for the Reform of Marijuana Laws
Norpramin (desipramine), 139, 147, 149–150
North Africa, 240
North Carolina, 21
Nortriptyline, 169
NSAIDs (nonsteroidal anti-inflammatory drugs), 109–110, 131. See also Ibuprofen
Nutt, Dana, 27–28
Nutt, Keith, 28–32

Ocupress (carteolol), 66
Ocusert (pilocarpine), 46, 50–51, 58, 59, 63
Oglesby, Carl, 68–72
Ohio State Medical Society, 4
Oligodendroglioma, 118
Ondansetron (Zofran), 24–25, 36, 38, 42, 169, 254
Opiates, 7, 209, 210–214, 245, 268, 271
Opioid narcotics, 109, 112, 114, 201
Opioids, 14, 76, 94, 109, 110, 122, 214
Opium, 5, 10, 210, 268
Organic Personality Disorder, Aggressive Type, 196
O'Shaughnessy, W. B., 4, 5
Osler, William, 6, 182
Osteoarthritis, 127–129. See also Arthritis
Ovarian cysts, 137
Oxycodone, 76, 175

Pain, 109–123, 260, 262. See also Phantom limb pain
Palacky University (Olomuc, Czechoslovakia), 172
Panama Canal Zone, 195
Papi, Michael, 155–157
Paraplegia and quadriplegia, 94–100
Parents for a Drug-Free America, 157–158

Parker, C. S., 141
Parnate (tranylcypromine), 139
Paroxetine (Paxil), 140
Partnership for a Drug-Free America, 42
Paufler, Greg, 81–86, 232
Paxil (paroxetine), 140
Pemoline (Cylert), 177
Penicillin, 172, 227, 253, 254, 255
Pentazocine (Talwin), 13–14
Perception enhancement, 279, 281–282
Percodan, 76, 175
Perphenazine (Trilafon), 155
Phantom limb pain, 200–202
Phenelzine (Nardil), 140
Phenobarbital, 67, 68, 72, 73, 74, 76,
    125, 165, 166
Phenothiazines, 241
Phenytoin (Dilantin), 67, 68, 72, 73, 74,
    76, 118, 120, 121, 175
Phos-Lo, 170
Phospholine iodide, 51, 60
Physical therapy, 175
Physicians, 20–21, 232–233, 260
Physicians' Association for AIDS Care, 13
Physostigmine, 87
Pierson, Lynn, 18, 19
Pilocarpine (Ocusert), 46, 50–51, 58,
    59, 63
Platinol (cisplatin), 23, 28, 36, 37, 38
PMS. See Premenstrual syndrome
Pneumonia, bacterial, 248–249
Police, 262; Los Angeles, 46–47
Pond, D. A., 141
Post-partum psychosis, 5
Post-traumatic stress disorder (PTSD),
    198–200
Potassium depletion, 84
Potency. See Dosage: potency; Mari-
    huana: potency
Prednisone, 80, 83, 124, 170, 188, 192
Pregnancy, 137–138, 249–250
Premenstrual syndrome, 127, 135–137.
    See also Cramps
Primidone (Mysoline), 67, 72, 73, 74,
    76

Prochlorperazine (Compazine), 24, 28,
    33, 105, 169, 170, 187, 222
Proctor, R. C., 210
Promethazine, 105
Propine (dipivefrine), 63
Propoxyphene (Darvon), 98, 122, 125,
    184
Propranolol, 87, 228
Propulsid (cisapride), 189, 190
Prostaglandin, 96
Protease inhibitors, 108
Protriptyline (Vivactil), 146
Prozac (fluoxetine), 105, 137, 140, 143,
    147, 148, 149, 175, 197, 199, 217,
    274
Pruritus, 131–135, 232
Pseudopseudohypoparathyroidism,
    111–118
Pseudotumor cerebri, 191–193, 260
Psoriasis, 104
Psychedelic drugs, 242–243, 267
Psychoactive drugs, 13, 180, 267–269,
    270–272, 275
Psychosis, 8. See also Post-partum
    psychosis; Side effects: psychosis
Public Health Service, 22
Pulmonary system, 250–252
Pure Food and Drug Act (1906), 269,
    270
Pyrahexyl, 210

Quadriplegia. See Paraplegia and quadri-
    plegia

Rabies, 4
Ramsey, H. H., 67
Randall, Robert, 21, 48–58, 232, 251–
    252
Ranitidine (Zantac), 105, 119, 146, 169,
    188
Raynaud's phenomenon, 181, 182, 183
Recreational use, 8, 37, 101, 266
Reefer Madness (film), 8, 195
Reglan (metoclopramide), 189, 190, 222
Religious freedom defense, 15

Reproductive system, 248, 249–250. See also Sexual function

Research, 256–257: state programs, 17–18, 25, 44, 262

Respiratory system. See Pulmonary system

Retching, 24, 28, 33. See also Vomiting

Retin-A (tretinoin), 228

Reynolds, J. R., 5–6, 135, 221

Rheumatic diseases, 3, 4, 5, 6, 126–131

Ritalin (methylphenidate), 143, 184, 193, 197–198

Robaxin (methocarbamol), 175

Rosenfeld, Irvin, 111–118

Ross, Karen, 118–122

Safer, Jeanne, 38

Safety: consumer, 272–273; of marihuana use, 6, 235, 254

San Francisco, 263, 265

San Francisco Buyers' Club, 265

Scheduled drugs. See Comprehensive Drug Abuse Prevention and Control Act

Schizophrenia, 178–181, 240, 241–242

Scientific Advisory Committee of the San Francisco Community Consortium, 257

Scleroderma (systemic sclerosis), 181–186

Scleroderma Association, 185

Seattle, 263

Seconal (secobarbital), 184, 235

Sedative properties. See Hypnotic properties

Seizures. See Epilepsy

Selective serotonin reuptake inhibitors. See SSRIs

Serotonin, 124, 126

Sertraline (Zoloft), 140, 197

Sexual function, 86, 88, 96, 99, 144, 147, 190, 249, 250

Sexual response, 11, 144, 161, 249, 250, 281, 282

Side effects, 19, 161, 234; acute effects,

235–243; anxiety, 239–40; chronic effects, 243–252; flashbacks, 242–243; hallucinations, 240, 242; high, 238; mental deterioration, 245; operating machinery, 236–238; personality changes, 247; psychosis, 240–241; stepping-stone theory, 245; toxic delirium, 242. See also Anxiety; Pulmonary system; Reproductive system; Toxicity; UKU Side Effect Rating Scale; and specific drugs, substances, and conditions

Skin disorders, 3, 218. See also Dermatitis

Sleep. See Hypnotic properties

Snakebite, 3

Soma (carisoprodol), 175

Sopor (methaqualone), 112, 113, 118

South Africa, 3

South America, 3

Southeast Asia, 3

Spasmodic torticollis. See Dystonias

Spastic disorders, 262

Spear, Donald, 131–135, 232

Sperm count, 249

Spleen, 262n

SSRIs (selective serotonin reuptake inhibitors), 137, 139. See also Paroxetine (Paxil); Prozac (fluoxetine); Sertraline (Zoloft)

Stamate, Byron, 219–221

Staphylococcus, 172, 248

Steroids, 94, 164. See also Corticosteroids

Stillbirths, 249. See also Childbirth

Stockings, G. T., 141

Streptococcus, 248

Stroup, Keith, 54

Sulfasalazine, 186

Sumatriptan (Imitrex), 124

Synhexyl, 2

Synthetic thyroid hormone, 143

Systemic sclerosis. See Scleroderma

Taft, Harris, 32–35

Tagamet (cimetidine), 184

Talshir, Debbi, 89–91

Talwin (pentazocine), 13–14
Tegretol (carbamazepine), 67, 141, 153
Tennessee, 213
Terminal illness, 5, 222–225, 263
Testicular cancer, 28, 36, 37
Testosterone, 249
Tetanus, 4, 5
Tetrahydrocannabinol. *See* THC
Texas, 204
Thacore, V. R., 241
THC (tetrahydrocannabinol), 2–3, 87,
    110, 126, 141–142, 164–165, 172,
    235–237, 249, 256; delta-1-, 2; delta-
    8-, 27, 94, 173; delta-9-, 21, 27,
    43–44, 94, 173, 178; immunosuppres-
    sive effects, 94; oral, 100; synthetic,
    18, 19, 55, 141. *See also* Congeners;
    Dronabinol; Marihuana: smoked vs.
    oral THC; Marinol; Nabilone
Theophylline, 165–166, 167
Thompson, L. J., 210
Thorazine (Chlorpromazine), 124, 222
3,4-methylenedioxymethamphetamine
    (MDMA), 16
3TC (lamivudine), 108
Tic douloureux, 6
Tilden's solution, 44
Timoptic (timolol), 46, 63
Tinnitus, 193–195
Tobacco, 11, 48, 209, 244
Tofranil (imipramine), 139, 145, 149,
    184, 228
Tolectin (tolmetin), 130
Tolerance. *See individual drugs and
    substances*
Tolmetin (Tolectin), 130
Toxicity, 24, 92, 165, 235–236, 254
Tranquilizers, 132, 153, 212
Tranxene (clorazepate), 74
Tranylcypromine (Parnate), 139
Trazodone (Desyrel), 92, 148, 175
Tretinoin (Retin-A), 228
Tricyclics, 139, 140, 142, 143, 147
Trihexyphenidyl (Artane), 175
Trilafon (perphenazine), 155

Turkestan, 3
Tylenol. *See* Acetaminophen

UKU Side Effect Rating Scale, 179–180
Ulcer, 6
Underground Cannabis Buyers' Club,
    265
United Nations Single Convention on
    Narcotic Substances, 14
United States, 246–247; Army, 195;
    Congress, 8, 13, 258; Department of
    Defense, 199; Department of Justice,
    14; federal government, 54, 57–58,
    256–258, 263, 266–267, 269–270;
    First Circuit Court of Appeals, 16;
    marihuana in, 2, 4; Second Circuit
    Court of Appeals, 14; Supreme Court,
    65
United States Dispensatory (1854), 4
United States Pharmacopoeia and
    National Formulary, 8
University of California at Los Angeles,
    46; Jules Stein Eye Institute, 55, 57
University of California at San Francisco,
    257
University of Göttingen (Germany), 87
University of Iowa, 110
University of Miami, 60
University of Mississippi, 21
University of Virginia Medical College,
    113
Upjohn Company, 228
Urinalysis. *See* Drug testing

Vaccinations, 272
Valium (diazepam), 74, 76, 80–81, 84,
    85, 87, 94, 96, 127, 132, 149, 175,
    179, 184, 228, 238, 244
Valporic acid (Depakote), 67, 141, 153
Vasodilan (isoxsuprine), 184
Venereal diseases, 3, 4. *See also* Gonor-
    rhea
Vicodin, 175
Victoria (queen of England), 4, 135
Violence, 8, 195–198, 274

Vitamins, 188
Vivactil (protriptyline), 146
Volstead Act (1919), 269
Vomiting, 18, 19, 21, 24–30, 33–35,
    43–44, 222–224, 259

WAMM (Wo•Men's Alliance for Medical
    Marihuana), 76
Wellbutrin (bupropion), 148, 159
Wilmer Eye Institute (Johns Hopkins
    University), 56
Winthrop, Roger, 29
Wo•Men's Alliance for Medical Mari-
    huana (WAMM), 76
Woodward, W. C., 8–10
Wrigley, F. W., 141

Xalatan (latanoprost), 46, 66
Xanax (alprazolam), 119, 120, 149, 238,
    277

Young, Bill, 210–214
Young, Francis L., 15–16
Young, Robert, 29

Zantac (ranitidine), 105, 119, 146, 169,
    188
Zarontin (ethosuximide), 67
Zidovudine. *See* AZT
Zofran (ondansetron), 24–25, 36, 38,
    42, 169, 254
Zoloft (sertraline), 140, 197

Marihuana, The Forbidden Medicine

Revised and Expanded Edition

Lester Grinspoon, M.D. and James B. Bakalar

In this important and timely book, two eminent researchers describe the medical benefits of marihuana, explain why its use has been forbidden, and argue for its full legalization to make it available to all patients who need it. Highly praised when it was first published in 1993, the book has been expanded to include new examples of the ways that marihuana alleviates symptoms of cancer chemotherapy, multiple sclerosis, osteoarthritis, glaucoma, AIDS, and depression, as well as symptoms of such less common disorders as Crohn's disease, diabetic gastroparesis, and post-traumatic stress disorder.

Praise for the first edition:

"Grinspoon and Bakalar have provided **a valuable compendium of marihuana's beneficial properties.** . . . This book is valuable for its breadth of first-person accounts of beneficial effects of marihuana smoking in physically and emotionally distressed individuals." —Rick J. Strassman, M.D., *Journal of the American Medical Association*

"Cogent and convincing arguments for the legalization of marihuana and its pharmacologically active components. . . . This book provides an excellent overview of the subject from a medical perspective." — Robert M. Swift, M.D., Ph.D., *New England Journal of Medicine*

"A very important book. . . . It is highly recommended reading for anyone interested in the history, biomedical science, and public policy surrounding these most amazing plants." —David E. Presti and Richard Evans Schultes, *Journal of Psychoactive Drugs*

Lester Grinspoon, M.D., is associate professor of psychiatry at Harvard Medical School. **James B. Bakalar** is associate editor of the *Harvard Mental Health Letter* and a lecturer in law in the department of psychiatry at Harvard Medical School.

DATE DUE

JUN 0 4 2013